Anderson's
Dental Materials

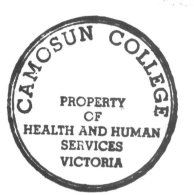

Anderson's Applied Dental Materials

J F McCabe

BSc PhD MRSC CChem
Senior Lecturer in Dental Materials Science
University of Newcastle upon Tyne

Sixth Edition

Blackwell Scientific Publications

OXFORD · LONDON · EDINBURGH

BOSTON · PALO ALTO · MELBOURNE

© 1956, 1961, 1965, 1967, 1972, 1976, 1985 by
Blackwell Scientific Publications
Editorial offices:
Osney Mead, Oxford, 0X2 OEL
8 John Street, London, WC1N 2ES
23 Ainslie Place, Edinburgh, EH3 6AJ
52 Beacon Street, Boston
    Massachusetts 02108, USA
744 Cowper Street, Palo Alto
    California 94301, USA
107 Barry Street, Carlton
    Victoria 3053, Australia

First published 1956
Second edition 1961
Reprinted 1965
Third edition 1967
Fourth edition 1972
Fifth edition 1976
Sixth edition 1985

Set by LP Printing Ltd
Hong Kong

Printed and bound in Great Britain by
Butler & Tanner Ltd,
Frome and London

DISTRIBUTORS

USA
    Blackwell Mosby Book Distributors
    11830 Westline Industrial Drive
    St Louis, Missouri 63141

Canada
    Blackwell Mosby Book Distributors
    120 Melford Drive, Scarborough
    Ontario M1B 2X4

Australia
    Blackwell Scientific Book Distributors
    31 Advantage Road, Highett
    Victoria 3190

British Library
Cataloguing in Publication Data

Anderson, John N.
    Anderson's applied dental materials.—6th ed.
    1.   Dental materials
    I. Title   II. McCabe, J.F.
    617.6′95   RK652.5

    ISBN 0-632-01217-X

Contents

Foreword

When I was writing the first edition of this book in 1955, dental materials was barely emerging as a scientific study. Much of the teaching and research was carried out by metallurgists, or by clinicians with a particular interest in the subject. I little thought that almost thirty years later I would be handing over the writing of a sixth edition to a dental materials scientist with a worldwide reputation. Despite this change in authorship, the book will continue to deal with the application of science to the clinical and laboratory situations. I am flattered that my name is to continue in the title and wish Dr McCabe every success with this and future editions.

Emeritus Prof. J. N. Anderson
Baslow, Derbyshire, England.
June 1984

Preface

This textbook has been written mainly with the undergraduate dental student in mind, although it is hoped that many parts of the text may prove beneficial to dental technicians, dental surgery assistants and practicing dentists.

The layout is such that it should help various interested groups to isolate their areas of interest within the book. For example, Chaps. 1 and 2 are introductory chapters which deal with the science of dental materials and the ways in which materials are characterized and their properties determined. It is hoped that all readers will familiarize themselves with these two chapters.

Chaps. 3–13 deal with materials which are primarily handled by the dental technician in his laboratory. It is important that both dentist and dental technician have a sound knowledge of these materials.

Chaps. 14–19 deal with materials which may be considered to link directly the dental surgery with the laboratory. It is essential that both technician and dentist have a sound knowledge of these materials in order that they may converse over any problems which arise. Dental surgery assistants should also have a sound knowledge of these products, particularly with regard to the ways in which manipulative variables can affect the performance of the materials.

Chaps. 20–29 deal primarily with those materials which are used in the dental surgery. The dentist and his chairside assistant should have a good knowledge of these materials and particularly the ways in which manipulative variables can affect the properties of the materials and hence the success or failure of the treatment.

The main difficulty experienced in planning this book was deciding what to include and what to leave out. It was decided to include only those materials which are used, directly or indirectly, for the production of restorations, appliances or prostheses. Using this definition, gypsum is classified as a dental material because it is often used for constructing models or dies during the production of dentures or cast metal restorations. Radiographic film, on the other hand, is used in diagnosis, but not in the production of restorations etc., and is therefore not classified as a dental material for the purposes of this book.

Likewise denture cleansers and toothpastes are not considered as dental materials for the purposes of this book and no chapters have been included on these subjects. When such materials are known to have an effect on the properties of *bona fide* dental materials, however, they are given due regard and discussed in the section relating to the materials being affected.

Acknowledgements

I am grateful to many people who have helped and encouraged me during the production of this book. I owe a particular debt of gratitude to John Anderson, whose 'Applied Dental Materials' has been a standard text for many years and it is fitting that his name should appear in the title of this book. When Professor Anderson expressed a wish not to continue producing 'Applied Dental Materials' following his retirement from the University of Dundee, I was delighted that Blackwell Scientific Publications offered me the chance of writing a new book to fill the vacuum.

I am grateful to many friends and colleagues who have offered much help, advice and constructive criticism which hopefully has helped to ensure the accuracy and clinical relevance of much of the data and information enclosed within these pages. I would particularly like to thank the following colleagues who have willingly read and commented on various chapters within the book:

Mr T. Cowell, Mr I. Geffner, Mr M. Gross, Dr J.W. McCrorie, Mr I.D. Murray, Mr J.G. Robinson, Mr B.H. Smith and Mr A.W.G. Walls. In addition, I would like to thank Professor Roy Storer for his advice and encouragement during production of the manuscript.

My wife Pauline deserves special thanks for spending many hours in proof reading at both the manuscript and proof stages.

Sincere thanks are due to Miss G. Hunter, Departmental Secretary in the Prosthodontics Department, who carried out the onerous task of typing and sometimes re-typing the manuscript in a most efficient manner.

Finally, a special message of thanks goes to Mr B. Hill of the Dental Hospital Photographic Department who produced all the illustrations — a mammoth task which he took on with great enthusiasm.

Units of Measurement

The following table indicates units which are used in the text. Most are SI units, although there are some variations, particularly with regard to temperature which has been given in degrees Celcius, not degrees Kelvin ($K = °C + 273$).

Physical quantity or property	Unit	Name	Comments or explanations
Time	s	second	—
Length	m	metre	μm, mm, km, commonly used
Area	m^2	square metre	mm^2 also used
Volume	m^3	cubic metre	mm^3 also used
Mass	kg	kilogram	g also used
Temperature	°C	degrees Celcius	$K - 273°C*$
Acceleration	ms^{-2}	metre per square second	—
Force	N	newton	$kg\ ms^{-2}$
Stress or pressure	Pa	pascal	$Pa = Nm^{-2}$ MPa or GPa also commonly used
Viscosity	Pas	pascal seconds	Nsm^{-2}
Energy, work or heat	J	joule	$J = Nm$ kJ, MJ commonly used

* K is strictly the correct SI unit of temperature.

Prefixes used before units refer to constant by which the quantity must be multiplied e.g. $\mu = 10^{-6}$, $m = 10^{-3}$, $k = 10^3$, $M = 10^6$, $G - 10^9$.

Science of Dental Materials

1.1 Introduction

The science of dental materials involves a study of the composition and properties of materials and the way in which they interact with the environment in which they are placed. The selection of materials for any given application can thus be undertaken with confidence and sound judgement.

The dentist spends much of his professional career handling materials and the success or failure of many forms of treatment depends upon the correct selection of materials possessing adequate properties, combined with careful manipulation.

It is no exaggeration to state that the dentist and dental technician have a wider variety of materials at their disposal than any other profession. Rigid polymers, elastomers, metals, alloys, ceramics, inorganic salts and composite materials are all com-monly encountered. Some examples are given in Fig. 1.1 along with some of their uses in dentistry.

This classification of materials embodies an enormous variation in material properties from hard, rigid materials at one extreme to soft, flexible products at the other.

Many dental materials are fixed permanently into the patient's mouth or are removed only intermit-tently for cleaning. Such materials have to with-stand the effects of a most hazardous environment. Temperature variations, wide variations in acidity or alkalinity and high stresses all have an effect on the durability of materials.

Normal temperature variations in the oral cavity lie between 32°C and 37°C depending on whether the mouth is open or closed. The ingestion of hot or cold food or drink however, extends this tem-

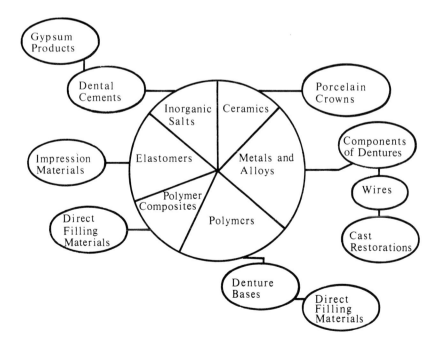

Fig. 1.1 Diagram indicating the wide variety of materials used in dentistry and some of their applications.

perature range from 0°C up to 70°C. The acidity or
alkalinity of fluids in the oral cavity as measured by
pH varies from around pH 4 to pH 8·5, whilst the
intake of acid fruit juices or alkaline medicaments
can extend this range from pH 2 to pH 11.

The load on one square millimetre of tooth or
restorative material can reach levels as high as
many kilograms indicating the demanding mechanical property requirements of some materials.

Many products, for example direct filling materials, are handled entirely by the dentist and his
chairside assistant and are rarely encountered by
the dental technician. Other materials are generally
associated with the work of the dental laboratory
and in this case both technician and dentist require
a thorough knowledge of the materials in order that
they may communicate about selection, manipulation and any problems which arise. A third group
of materials link the dental surgery and the laboratory. The most obvious example of such products
is the impression materials. Whilst the latter are
under the direct control of the dentist it is essential
that the dental technician also has a sound knowledge of such materials.

1.2 Selection of dental materials

The process of materials selection should ideally
follow a logical sequence involving (1) analysis of
the problem, (2) consideration of requirements,
(3) consideration of available materials and their
properties, leading to (4) choice of material.
Evaluation of the success or failure of a material
may be used to influence future decisions on materials selection. This selection process is illustrated
in Fig. 1.2. Many experienced practitioners carry
out this sequence with no apparent effort since they
are able to call upon a wealth of clinical experience. However, when presented with new or
modified materials even the most experienced
dentist returns to a more formal type of selection
process based on the criteria mentioned.

Analysis The analysis of the situation requiring
selection of a material may seem obvious but it is of
paramount importance in some circumstances. An
incorrect decision may cause failure of the restoration or appliance. For example, when considering
the selection of a filling material it is important to
decide whether the restoration is to be placed in an
area of high stress. Will it be visible when the
patient smiles? Is the cavity deep or shallow?

These factors and many more must be evaluated
before attempting materials selection.

Requirements Having completed a thorough
analysis of the situation it is possible to develop a
list of requirements for a material to meet the
needs of that situation. For the example mentioned
in the previous section, it may be decided that a
filling material which matches tooth colour and is
able to withstand moderately high stresses without
fracture is required. Some tooth cavities are caused
by toothbrush/toothpaste abrasion. In this special
case the restorative material used should naturally
possess adequate resistance to dentifrice abrasion.
The list of requirements is infinitely variable,
although some general classifications can be made.

Available materials The consideration of available
materials, their properties and how these compare
with the requirements is carried out at two levels.
The dentist, faced with the immediate problem of
restoring the tooth of a patient in his surgery, must
choose from those materials on hand at the time.
Previous experience with materials in similar circumstances will be a major factor which influences
selection. On a wider scale, the practitioner is able
to consider the use of alternative materials or newly
developed products where these appear to offer a
solution to cases which have proved difficult with
his existing armoury of products. It is of paramount
importance that the practitioner keeps up to date
with developments in materials whilst taking a conservative approach towards adopting new products
for regular use in his surgery until they are properly
tested.

Choice of material Having compared the properties
of the available materials with the requirements, it
is possible to narrow the choice to a given generic
group of products. The final choice of material
brand is often a matter of personal preference on
the part of the dentist. Factors such as ease of
handling, availability and cost may play a part at
this stage of the selection process.

1.3 Evaluation of materials

As the number of available materials increases, it
becomes more and more important for the dentist
to be protected from unsuitable products or materials which have not been thoroughly evaluated.
It should be emphasized, however, that most manu-

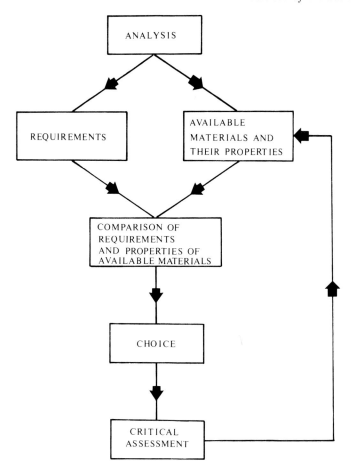

Fig. 1.2 Flow chart indicating a logical method of material selection.

facturers of dental materials operate an extensive quality assurance programme and materials are thoroughly tested before being released to the general practitioner.

Standard specifications Many standard specification tests, of both national and international standards organizations, are now available which effectively maintain quality levels for some dental materials. Such specifications normally give details for the testing of certain products, the method of calculating the results and the minimum permissible result which is acceptable. Although such specifications play a useful part they should not be seen as indicating total suitability since the tests carried out often do not cover critical aspects of the use of a material. For example, many materials fail by a fatigue mechanism in practice, but few specifica-

tions involve fatigue testing.

Laboratory evaluations Laboratory tests, some of which are used in standard specifications, can be used to indicate the suitability of certain materials. For example, a simple solubility test can indicate the stability of a material in aqueous media — a very important property for filling materials.

It is important that methods used to evaluate materials in the laboratory give results which can be correlated with clinical experience. For example, when upper dentures fracture along the midline they do so through bending. Hence a bending or transverse strength test is far more meaningful for these materials than a compression test.

Clinical trials Although laboratory tests can provide many important and useful data on materials, the ultimate test is the controlled clinical trial and the verdict of practitioners after a period of use in general practice. Many materials produce good results in the laboratory, only to be found lacking when subjected to clinical use. The majority of manufacturers carry out extensive clinical trials of new materials, normally in co-operation with a university or hospital department, prior to releasing a product for use by general practitioners.

2

Properties used to Characterize Materials

2.1 Introduction

Many factors must be taken into account when considering which properties are relevant to the successful performance of a material used in dentistry. The situation in which the material is to be used and the recommended technique for its manipulation define the properties which characterize the material. Laboratory tests used to evaluate materials often duplicate conditions which exist *in situ*. This is not always possible and sometimes not desirable since one aim of *in vitro* testing is to predict in a rapid laboratory test what may happen in the mouth over a number of months or years. Many tests used to evaluate dental materials involve the measurement of simple properties such as compressive strength or hardness which have been shown to correlate with clinical performance.

Many materials used in dentistry are supplied as two or more components which are mixed together and undergo a chemical reaction, during which the mechanical and physical properties may change

dramatically. For example, many impression materials are supplied as fluid pastes which begin to set when mixed together. The set material may be a rigid solid or a flexible rubber depending upon the chemical nature of the product.

The acceptance of such a product by the dentist depends upon the properties of the unmixed paste, the properties during mixing and setting and the properties of the set material (Fig. 2.1). This classification of properties applies to virtually all groups of materials.

Properties of unmixed materials Manufacturers formulate materials which give optimal performance as evaluated by their quality assurance programme and clinical trials. It is known however, that certain products deteriorate during storage and as a result may perform poorly. Such materials are said to have limited 'shelf life'. Some materials have an extended 'shelf life' if refrigerated during storage. One technique commonly employed to predict

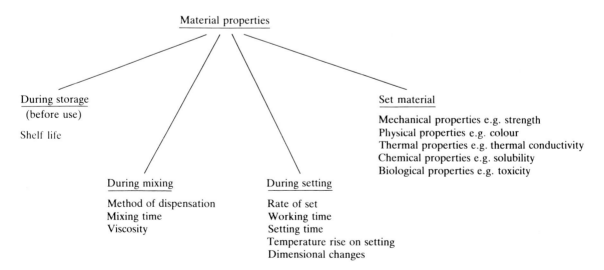

Fig. 2.1 An indication of the properties which are used to characterize dental materials.

stability is to carry out accelerated ageing by storing samples at elevated temperature, commonly 60°C, followed by evaluation of material properties.

Containers used for materials generally have a batch number stamped or printed onto them from which the date of manufacture can be obtained. Thus, for materials with limited shelf life it is possible to ascertain the date at which one would expect the properties to deteriorate.

Properties of materials during mixing, manipulation and setting Properties of materials during mixing, manipulation and setting are considered together since they mainly involve a consideration of rheological properties and the way in which these change as a function of time during setting.

For materials of two or more components which set by a chemical reaction, thorough mixing is essential in order to achieve homogenous distribution of properties throughout the material. The ease of mixing depends on factors such as the chemical affinity of the components, the viscosity, both of the components and the mixed material, the ambient temperature, the method of dispensation and the method of mixing.

Several methods of dispensation exist among materials used in dentistry. Some involve the mixing of powder and liquid components, others the mixing of two pastes, while others involve paste and liquid components. When the mixing of two pastes is required, the manufacturer often gives a good colour contrast between the two pastes. The achievement of a thorough mix of the two components can be judged by the attainment of a homogeneous colour with no streaks. When powder and liquid or paste and liquid are mixed, the achievement of a thorough mix is less certain. The components are mixed for a recommended time and/or until a recommended consistency is reached.

A growing number of materials are mixed mechanically. This method removes uncertainty and gives a more reproducible result.

The use of encapsulated materials which are mixed mechanically is becoming very popular. These offer the dual advantages of easier and more reproducible mixing coupled with pre-set proportions of components within the capsules.

Certain products have specific manipulative requirements which will be referred to later. For many applications, materials should be in a relatively fluid state at the time they are introduced into the patient's mouth but should undergo rapid setting involving a change to a more rigid or rubbery form. From the commencement of mixing, two important times can be defined which have an important bearing on the acceptability of materials. The first is the *working time*, defined as the time available for mixing and manipulating a material. For example, an impression material should be seated in the mouth before the end of the working time otherwise setting will have proceeded sufficiently for the viscosity to have increased considerably. The other time which characterizes setting is the *setting time*. This, like working time, is to some extent arbitrary since it is defined as the time taken for a material to have reached a certain level of rigidity or elasticity. It is known that many materials continue setting for a considerable time after the apparent setting and optimum properties may not be achieved until several hours later.

Properties of the set material The properties of the unmixed material and those during mixing and setting are important and may influence the practitioner's selection. Generally, it is the properties of the set material which indicate the suitability of a product for any application. For example, in the case of a filling material, the method of dispensation, viscosity of the mixed material, working time and setting time control the ease of handling of the product, but the durability of the material in the oral environment depends on factors such as strength, solubility, abrasion resistance etc. The properties of the set material can be conveniently divided into the following categories: mechanical properties, thermal properties, chemical properties, biological properties and miscellaneous other physical properties. Naturally, the properties relevant to any one material will depend on the application.

2.2 Mechanical properties

Most applications of materials in dentistry have a minimum mechanical property requirement. For example, certain materials should be sufficiently strong to withstand biting forces without fracture. Others should be rigid enough to maintain their shape under load. Such properties of materials are generally characterized by the stress−strain relationship which is readily obtained by using a testing machine of the type shown in Fig. 2.2.

Before considering the various types of experiment which can be carried out and the relevance of the data obtained, it is necessary to define the

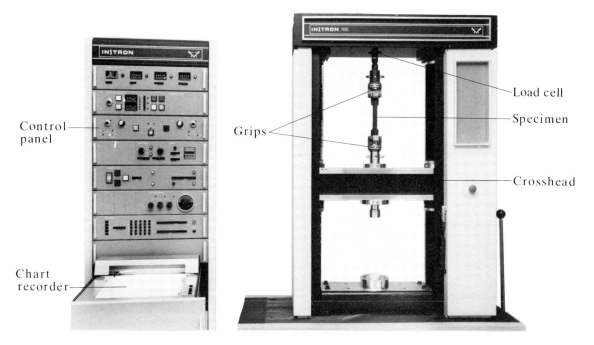

Fig. 2.2 Testing machine used for evaluating mechanical properties. Photograph shows the machine in the 'tensile mode'.

terms stress and strain.

Stress When an external force is applied to a body or specimen of material under test, an internal force, equal in magnitude but opposite in direction, is set up in the body. For simple compression or tension the stress is given by the expression — Stress = F/A where F is the applied force and A the cross-sectional area (Fig. 2.3). A stress resisting a compressive force is referred to as a compressive stress and that resisting a tensile force a tensile stress.

Tensile and compressive stresses, along with shear, are the three simple examples of stress which form the basis of all other more complex stress patterns. The unit of stress is the pascal (Pa). This is the stress resulting from a force of 1 newton (N) acting upon one square metre of surface.

One test method commonly used for dental materials is the three-point bending test or transverse test (Fig. 2.4).

When an external force is applied to the mid-point of the test beam the stresses can be resolved as shown. The numerical value of stress is given by the expression

$$\text{Stress} = \frac{3FL}{2bd^2}$$

where L is the distance between the supports, b is the width of the specimen and d its depth.

When a cylinder of a brittle material is compressed across a diameter as shown in Fig. 2.5a, a tensile stress is set up in the specimen, the value of the stress being given by

$$\text{Stress} = \frac{2F}{\pi\,DT} \text{ at the axis of the cylinder,}$$

where F is the applied force, D the diameter of the cylinder and T the length of the cylinder. This type of test is referred to as a diametral compressive tensile test and is commonly used when conventional tensile testing is difficult to carry out due to the brittle nature of the test material. For non-brittle materials the equation used to calculate stress breaks down due to the increased area of contact between the testing machine platen and the material under test (Fig. 2.5b).

Fracture stress — strength There is a limit to the value of applied force which a body, or specimen of material, can withstand without fracturing. The stress at fracture is normally used to characterize the strength of a material. In a tensile test, the fracture stress is referred to as the tensile strength of a material whilst a compression test gives a value of compressive strength. The diametral compress-

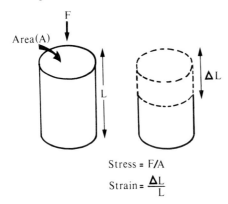

Stress = F/A

Strain = $\frac{\Delta L}{L}$

(a) Compression

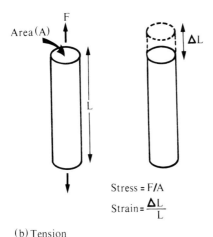

Stress = F/A

Strain = $\frac{\Delta L}{L}$

(b) Tension

Fig. 2.3 Diagram indicating how the magnitudes of (a) compressive and (b) tensile stresses and strains are calculated.

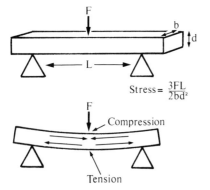

Stress = $\frac{3FL}{2bd^2}$

Fig. 2.4 Diagrammatic representation of a 3-point bending test or transverse test. Bending of the beam introduces both tensile and compressive stresses.

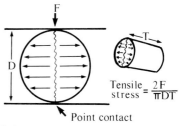

Tensile stress = $\frac{2F}{\pi DT}$

(a) Brittle material

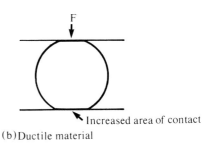

(b) Ductile material

Fig. 2.5 Diametral compressive test for (a) a brittle material and (b) a ductile material.

ive tensile test gives a value for tensile strength.

In the case of a bending test, fracture is normally initiated from the side of the specimen which is in tension. The bending stress at fracture, often called the flexural stress, is closely related to the tensile strength.

Strain The application of an external force to a body or test specimen results in a change in dimension of that body. For example, when a tensile force is applied the body undergoes an extension, the magnitude of which depends on the applied force and the properties of the material. The numerical value of strain is given by the expression

$$\text{Strain} = \frac{\text{Change in length}}{\text{Original length}}$$

Thus strain, which has no physical dimensions, can be seen as a measure of the fractional change in length caused by an applied force (Fig. 2.3). The strain may be recoverable, that is the material will return to its original length after removal of the applied force, or the material may remain deformed, in which case the strain is non-recoverable. A third possibility is that the strain may be partially recoverable. The extent to which the strain is recovered is a function of the elastic properties of materials.

Stress—strain relationship Stress and strain, as defined in the previous sections, are not independent and unrelated properties, but are closely related and may be seen as an example of cause and effect. The application of an external force, producing a stress within a material, results in a change in dimension or strain within the body.

The relationship between stress and strain is often used to characterize the mechanical properties of materials. Such data are generally obtained using a mechanical testing machine (Fig. 2.2) which enables strain to be measured as a function of stress and recorded automatically. Modern machines are capable of either increasing strain at a given rate and measuring the stress or increasing stress at a given rate and measuring the strain. Other applications, including fatigue testing, will be covered later.

For the simplest type of tensile or compression test, the graph displayed on the pen recorder would be as shown in Fig. 2.6.

It can be seen that in this example there is a linear relationship between stress and strain up to the point P. Further increases in stress cause proportionally greater increases in strain until the material fractures at point T. The stress corresponding to point T is the fracture stress. In a tensile test this gives a value of *tensile strength*, whilst in a compression test a value of *compressive strength* is obtained. The value of stress which corresponds to the limit of proportionality, P, is referred to as the *proportional limit*.

Point E is the *elastic limit*. This corresponds to the stress beyond which strains are not fully recovered. Hence, it is the maximum stress which a material can withstand without undergoing some permanent deformation. The elastic limit is difficult to characterize experimentally since it requires a series of experiments in which the stress is gradually increased then released and observations on elastic recovery made.

As a consequence of these experimental difficulties the *proportional limit* is often used to give an approximation to the value of the *elastic limit*. Hence, when a material is reported as having a high value of proportional limit it indicates that a sample of the material is more likely to withstand applied stress without permanent deformation.

A practical example of a situation in which a high proportional limit is required is in connectors of partial dentures. Such connectors should not undergo permanent deformation if they are to retain their shape. A material such as cobalt−chromium alloy which has a high value of proportional limit is popular for this application since it can withstand high stresses without being permanently distorted.

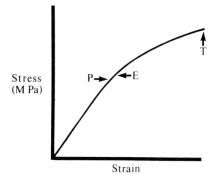

Fig. 2.6 Typical stress−strain graph obtained from a simple compressive or tensile test.

The slope of the straight-line portion of the stress−strain graph gives a measure of the *modulus of elasticity* defined as:

$$\text{Modulus of elasticity} = \frac{\text{Stress}}{\text{Strain}}$$

This has units of stress. The choice of nomenclature for this property is somewhat unfortunate since it, in fact, gives an indication of the rigidity of a material and *not* its elasticity. A steep slope, giving a high modulus value, indicates a rigid material, whilst a shallow slope, giving a low modulus value,

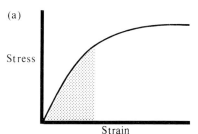

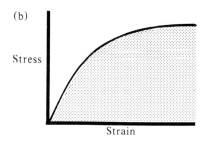

Fig. 2.7 The area under a stress−strain graph may be used to calculate either (a) resilience or (b) toughness.

indicates a flexible material. Whereas it may be advantageous for an impression material to be flexible it is essential for a restorative material to be rigid.

The value of strain recorded between points E and T indicates the degree of permanent deformation which can be imparted to a material up to the point of fracture. For a tensile test this gives an indication of *ductility* whilst for a compressive test it indicates *malleability*. Hence, a ductile material can be bent or stretched by a considerable amount without fracture whereas a malleable material can be hammered into a thin sheet. A property often used to give an indication of ductility is the *elongation at fracture*. Alloys used to form wires must show a high degree of ductility since they are extended considerably during the production process. In addition, clasps of dentures constructed from ductile alloys can be altered by bending.

The malleability of stainless steel is utilized when forming a denture base by the swaging technique. This involves the adaptation of a sheet of stainless steel over a preformed cast.

The area beneath the stress—strain curve yields some important information about test materials (Fig. 2.7). The area beneath the curve up to the elastic limit, Fig. 2.7a, gives a value of *resilience*, the units being those of energy. Resilience may be defined as the energy absorbed by a material in undergoing elastic deformation up to the elastic limit. A high value of resilience is one parameter often used to characterize elastomers. Such materials which may, for example, be used to apply a cushioned lining to a hard denture base are able to absorb considerable amounts of energy without being permanently distorted. The energy is stored and released when the material springs back to its original shape after removal of the applied stress.

The total area under the stress—strain graph, Fig. 2.7b, gives an indication of *toughness*. This again has units of energy and may be defined as the total amount of energy which a material can absorb up to the point of fracture. A material capable of absorbing large quantities of energy is termed a *tough material*. The opposite of toughness is brittleness. This is, naturally, an important property for many dental materials. Its measurement, for example in a transverse test, depends on factors such as the speed with which the stress is increased and the presence of small imperfections in the specimen surface from which cracks can propagate. In order to prevent the latter effect from influencing the

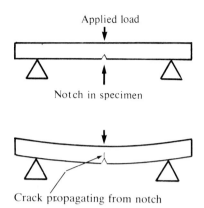

Fig. 2.8 Notched specimens are often used in tests of toughness in order to overcome the effects of surface imperfections in specimens.

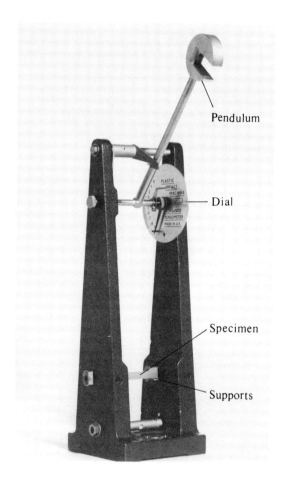

Fig. 2.9 Swinging pendulum machine used for measuring impact strength.

results, notched specimens are often used (Fig. 2.8). When the stress is increased rapidly in such a test it may be termed an *impact test* and the important practical property obtained is the *impact strength* which is often quoted in units of energy. For this type of test the machine shown in Fig. 2.2 is often not capable of increasing stress rapidly enough and a swinging pendulum impact testing device is commonly used (Fig. 2.9). The position reached by the pendulum after fracturing the specimen gives a measure of the energy absorbed by the specimen during fracture. Impact strength is an important property for acrylic denture base materials which have a tendency to fracture if accidentally dropped onto a hard surface.

Fig. 2.10 gives examples of various types of stress–strain graphs which may be encountered, along with an explanation of the way in which the graphs can be used to characterize materials.

Fatigue properties Many materials which are used as restoratives or dental prostheses are subjected to intermittent stresses over a long period of time — possibly many years. Although the stresses encountered may be far too small to cause fracture of a material when measured in a direct tensile, compressive or transverse test it is possible that, over a period of time, failure may occur by a fatigue process. This involves the formation of a microcrack at the surface, possibly caused by stress concentration at a surface fault or due to the shape of the restoration or prosthesis. This crack slowly propagates until fracture occurs. Final fracture often occurs at quite a low level of stress, a fact which often surprises patients who claim that their denture fractured when biting on soft food.

Fatigue properties may be studied in one of two ways. Firstly, it is possible to apply a cyclic stress at a given magnitude and frequency and to observe the number of cycles required for failure. The result is often referred to as the 'fatigue life' of a

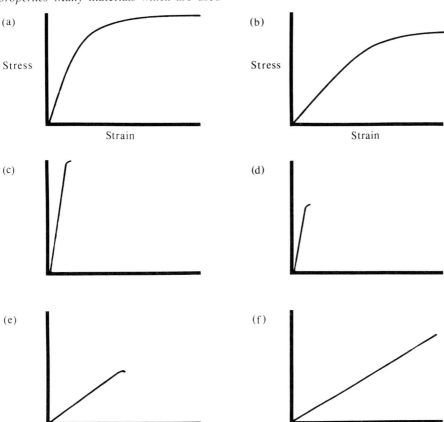

Fig. 2.10 Six different types of stress–strain graphs. These may be used to characterize materials as follows: (a) rigid, strong, tough, ductile; (b) flexible, tough; (c) rigid, strong, brittle; (d) rigid, weak, brittle; (e) flexible, weak, brittle; (f) flexible, resilient.

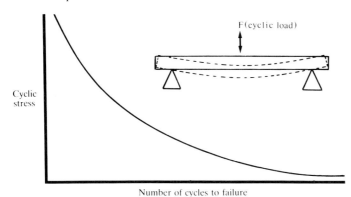

Fig. 2.11 Fatigue testing. Results are often given as a graph of cyclic stress versus number of cycles to failure. At smaller stress levels a greater number of cycles are required to cause fracture.

material. Another approach is to select a given number of stress cycles, say 10 000, and determine the value of the cyclic stress which is required to cause fracture within this number of cycles. The result in this case is referred to as the 'fatigue limit'. Both methods play an important part in materials evaluation. The most rigorous approach is to test many specimens at different cyclic stress levels and to determine the number of cycles to failure in each case. The result is then given in the form of a graph as shown in Fig. 2.11. As the applied cyclic stress increases, the number of cycles to failure decreases.

One of the most important factors involved in such tests is the quality of the specimen used in the test since faults introduced during preparation can drastically reduce both fatigue life and fatigue limit.

Abrasion resistance The oral cavity is a relatively harsh environment in which to place either a restoration or prosthesis. *Wear* can occur by one or more of a number of mechanisms, some of which may be considered to be of mechanical origin and others chemical. Wear caused by indenting and scratching of the surface by abrasive toothpastes or food is termed *abrasive wear* and the hardness of a material is often used to give an approximate indication of the resistance to this type of abrasion.

Wear due to intermittent stresses caused by, for example, tooth−restorative contacts where the degree of scratching may be minimal is termed *fatigue wear* and the fatigue life and fatigue limit mentioned in the previous section are thought to give a guide to the fatigue wear resistance.

In practice the position is not as clear cut as it would seem from the previous two paragraphs since most wear processes occur by a combination of two or more mechanisms. Consequently, laboratory experiments devised to measure wear rates of

dental materials often produce unconvincing or even misleading results.

The most important comparative information about the abrasion resistance values of different materials comes from well-controlled clinical trials.

Wear of certain materials can often be attributed to chemical degradation. Such processes are often referred to as erosion processes in order to distinguish them from the mechanical degradation involved in either abrasive wear or fatigue wear. Chemical properties, including erosion, will be discussed later.

Hardness The hardness of a material gives an indication of the resistance to penetration when indented by a hard asperity. The value of hardness, often referred to as the hardness number, depends on the method used for its evaluation. Generally, low values of hardness number indicate a soft material and vice versa.

Common methods used for hardness evaluation include Vickers, Knoop, Brinell and Rockwell. Vickers and Knoop both involve the use of diamond pyramid indentors. In the case of Vickers hardness, the diamond pyramid has a square base, whilst for Knoop hardness, one axis of the diamond pyramid is much larger than the other. The Brinell hardness test involves the use of a steel ball indentor producing an indentation of circular cross-section. Fig. 2.12 shows the types of indentation produced in test specimens. The hardness is a function of the diameter of the circle for Brinell hardness and the distance across the diagonal axes for Vickers and Knoop hardness. Allowance is naturally made for the magnitude of the applied loads.

Measurements are normally made using a microscope since the indentations are often too small to be seen with the naked eye. In the case of Rockwell hardness, a direct measurement of the depth

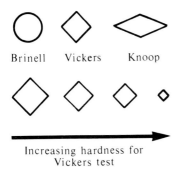

Brinell   Vickers   Knoop

Increasing hardness for
Vickers test

Fig. 2.12 Shapes of indentations produced by three types of hardness test. A decrease in the size of the indentation indicates a harder material.

of penetration of a conical diamond indentor is made. Table 2.1 shows Vickers hardness numbers for some common dental materials.

Hardness is often used to give an indication of the ability to resist scratching. Hence, acrylic materials are easily scratched because they are relatively soft whereas Co/Cr alloys are unlikely to become scratched because they are relatively hard. As a corollary to this, harder materials are more

difficult to polish by mechanical means.

Hardness is also used to give an indication of the abrasion resistance of a material, particularly where the wear process is thought to include scratching as in abrasive wear.

Elasticity and viscoelasticity The property of *yield stress* has previously been used to define the elastic range of a material. The yield stress is the value of stress beyond which the material becomes permanently distorted, that is, the strain is not recovered after the applied load is removed.

Although yield stress is an important property it does not, on its own, fully characterize the elastic properties of a material. Elastic properties are

Table 2.1 Vickers hardness numbers of some selected dental materials

Material	VHN
Enamel	350
Dentine	60
Acrylic resin	20
Dental amalgam	100
Porcelain	450
Co/Cr alloys	420

Fig. 2.13 Models used to represent (a) elastic materials, (b) plastic materials, and (c) and (d) viscoelastic materials.

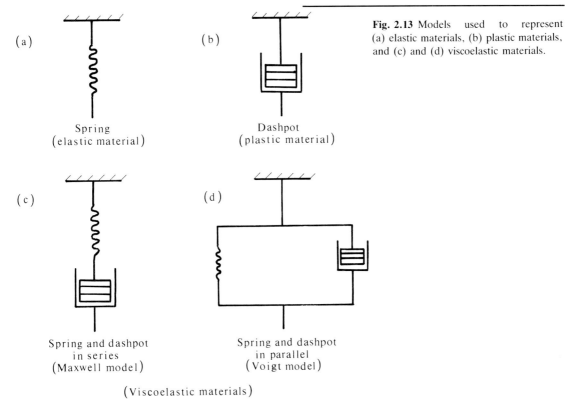

(a) Spring
(elastic material)

(b) Dashpot
(plastic material)

(c) Spring and dashpot
in series
(Maxwell model)

(d) Spring and dashpot
in parallel
(Voigt model)

(Viscoelastic materials)

(a)

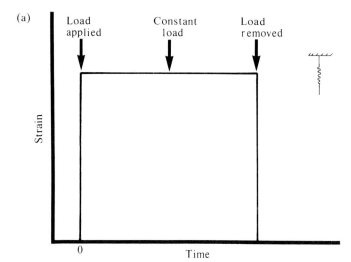

Fig. 2.14 Strain versus time graphs obtained for various types of model materials. (a) Elastic material, (b) plastic material, (c) viscoelastic material (Maxwell-type), (d) viscoelastic material (Voigt-type).

(b)

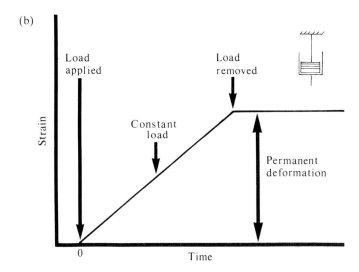

often defined in terms of the ability of a material to undergo *elastic recovery*. When a material undergoes full elastic recovery immediately after removal of an applied load it is *elastic*. If the recovery takes place slowly, or if a degree of *permanent deformation* remains, the material is said to be *viscoelastic*.

Models involving the use of springs and dashpots can be used to explain the elastic and viscoelastic behaviour of materials (Fig. 2.13). When a spring, which represents an elastic material, is fixed at one end and a load applied at the other it becomes instantaneously extended. When the load is removed it immediately recovers its original length, Fig. 2.14a.

When a load is applied to a dashpot, which represents a viscous material, it opens slowly, strain being a function of the *time* for which the load is applied, Fig. 2.14b. When the load is removed the dashpot remains open and no recovery occurs.

For the material behaving as a spring and dashpot in series (Maxwell model), application of a load causes the spring to be extended instantaneously followed by slow opening of the dashpot, Fig. 2.14c. On removal of the load the spring recovers but the dashpot remains permanently distorted. The magnitude of the distortion depends on the *applied load* and the *time* for which the load is applied.

For the material behaving as a spring and dash-

(c)

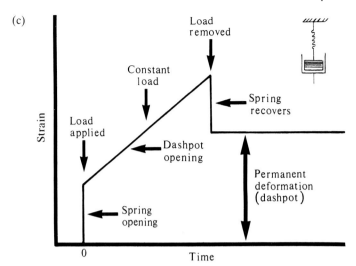

(d)

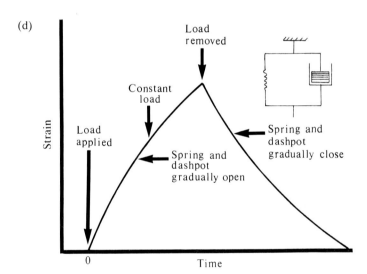

pot in parallel (Voigt model), application of load causes slow opening of the spring under the damping effect of the dashpot, Fig. 2.14d. Following removal of the load the dashpot and spring slowly recover to their original state under the elastic influence of the spring and the damping influence of the dashpot. The time taken to recover is a function of the *applied load* and the *time* of application of the load.

Many viscoelastic materials used in dentistry behave like a combination of the Voigt and Maxwell models (Fig. 2.15). Such materials show an instantaneous increase in strain due to the spring (A) followed by a gradual increase in strain as the dashpot (B) and spring/dashpot (C/D) system open.

On removal of the load the spring (A) recovers instantaneously followed by gradual recovery of the spring/dashpot (C/D). Some permanent distortion remains as a consequence of the dashpot (B). Again, the magnitude of the permanent deformation is a function of the *applied load* and the *time* of application.

This type of behaviour has important practical significance for many dental materials and particularly for 'elastic' impression materials. All such materials are viscoelastic to some extent and may become distorted when being removed over undercuts. The permanent deformation depends on the applied load, which in this case is a function of the force required to remove the impression from the

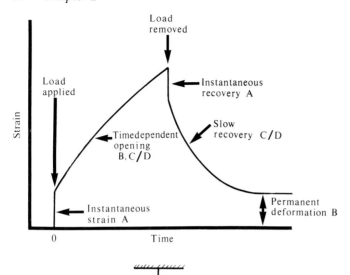

Fig. 2.15 Universal model which can be used to explain the viscoelastic properties of most materials.

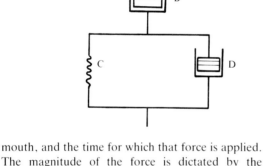

mouth, and the time for which that force is applied. The magnitude of the force is dictated by the modulus of elasticity of the material, its thickness and the severity of the undercuts.

Creep and *stress relaxation* are two other phenomena which can be explained using the viscoelasticity models.

Creep involves a gradual increase in strain under the influence of a constant applied load similar to that which takes place in the Maxwell model (Fig. 2.13c). Stress relaxation involves the 'application of a constant strain'. Under such conditions the stress decreases as a function of time for Maxwell-type viscoelastic materials. Although stress relaxation experiments can be used to classify materials, creep tests have more practical significance for dental materials. Such tests are relatively simple to carry out. A constant load is applied to a test specimen in either compression or tension. The

strain or creep is measured as a function of time. Dynamic creep tests are also carried out in which the load is applied at regular intervals and the change in the value of strain measured as a function of the number of loading cycles.

Values of creep obtained by such techniques are particularly important for dental amalgam. It is thought that creep is a precursor to fracture at the edge of the filling and hence failure for such materials.

Stress relaxation is a measure of decreasing stress at constant strain. It is not of direct relevance for most dental applications.

2.3 Rheological properties
Rheology is the study of the flow or deformation of materials. The term can be applied to both solids

and liquids and in the case of solids or elastomers involves the use of elasticity and viscoelasticity theory mentioned in Section 2.2. A study of the rheological properties of liquids and pastes normally involves the measurement of viscosity and the determination of the way in which this varies with factors such as rate of shear and time.

By definition viscosity (η) is given by the equation

$$\eta = \frac{\text{Shear stress } (\hat{6})}{\text{Shear rate } (E)}$$

The phenomena of *shear stress* and *shear rate* can be visualized by considering the extrusion of a fluid material from a syringe (Fig. 2.16). When the material is extruded at a constant rate the shear stress is related to the pressure required to depress the barrel of the syringe, whereas the shear rate is a function of the flow rate. Thus, a material of low viscosity requires only a low pressure to produce a high flow rate, whereas a more viscous material may require a high pressure to produce a relatively small rate of flow.

Further characterization of the rheological properties of materials is obtained by reference to the equation

$$\text{Shear stress} = K \,(\text{Shear rate})^{n}$$

where K and n are constants. The constant n is referred to as the *flow index*. For the simplest case, where $n = 1$, the shear stress is directly proportional to shear rate and the viscosity of the material is constant and independent of shear rate. Materials which behave in this way are referred to as *Newtonian fluids*.

When the flow index value is less than unity an increase in shear rate produces a less than proportionate increase in shear stress. Thus the viscosity is effectively decreased with increasing shear rate. Such materials are referred to as being *pseudoplastic*. When the flow index value is greater than unity an increase in shear rate produces a more than proportionate increase in shear stress, thus effectively increasing viscosity. Such materials are said to be *dilatant*.

Fig. 2.16 illustrates the result which may be obtained for Newtonian, pseudoplastic and dilatant materials when viscosity is measured as a function of shear rate. For dental materials, Newtonian and pseudoplastic behaviour are commonly encountered, whereas dilatancy is rare. The rheological properties are important for many different materials since they often control the ease of use.

Some materials exhibit so-called Bingham characteristics. Here, a finite stress, sometimes referred to as the yield stress of the substance, is required in order to cause the material to flow. Once the yield stress is exceeded the material may behave as a Newtonian, pseudoplastic or dilatant

Fig. 2.16 The rheological properties of fluids and pastes can be represented by the extrusion of materials from a syringe.

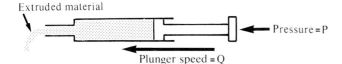

Extruded material

Pressure = P

Plunger speed = Q

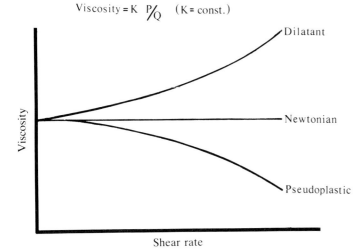

Viscosity = K P/Q (K = const.)

Dilatant

Newtonian

Pseudoplastic

Viscosity

Shear rate

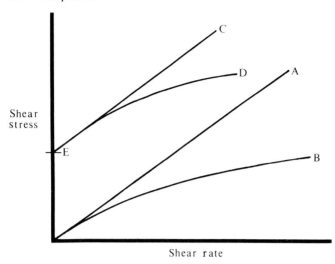

Shear stress

E

Shear rate

Fig. 2.17 Shear stress—shear rate plots of four materials. Two (A and B) have no yield stress whilst the other two (C and D) exhibit a yield stress of value E.

fluid. In Fig. 2.17 curve A represents the behaviour of a normal Newtonian fluid, curve B the behaviour of a normal pseudoplastic fluid, curve C the behaviour of a material with a yield stress (value E) followed by Newtonian behaviour and curve D the behaviour of a material with a yield stress followed by pseudoplastic behaviour.

Viscosity values of materials are temperature-dependent, an increase in temperature generally causing a significant reduction in viscosity.

Time-dependence of viscosity (*working times and setting times*) Many materials used in dentistry involve the mixing of two components, thus initiating a chemical reaction which causes the material to change from a fluid to a rigid solid or elastomer. The initial viscosity of the mixed material often governs its ease of handling. The rate at which the viscosity increases as a function of time is of equal importance. Manipulation becomes impossible when viscosity has increased beyond a certain point. The time taken to reach that point is the *working time* of the material.

Fig. 2.18 shows a typical plot of viscosity against time for a material setting by a chemical reaction (curve A). The material may become unmanageable when it reaches a viscosity value of V_1, thus the material has a working time of T_1. Curve B is the plot of a material for which the viscosity does not begin to increase until the time T_2 and the viscosity has not reached V_1 until the time T_3. Thus the working time for this material is considerably longer than that for material A. The shape of curve B suggests that the chemical reaction involved in

setting has an induction period, probably produced by chemical retarders which manufacturers sometimes use to extend working times.

The other important time used to define setting characteristics is the *setting time*. This is related to the time taken for the material to reach its final set state or to develop properties which are considered adequate for that application. Methods used for measuring setting characteristics vary from one type of material to another. One convenient and commonly used method is resistance to penetration. Thus a material may be considered set when it is able to resist penetration by a probe of known weight and tip diameter (Fig. 2.19). It can be seen that in Fig. 2.19a the material is readily penetrated by the probe indicating that it has not set, whilst in Fig. 2.19b the probe is supported by the material, indicating that it is now set. As with most other methods of setting-time evaluation, this one is to some extent arbitrary in that the value obtained depends on the weight and tip diameter of the probe. ·

2.4 Thermal properties
Wide temperature fluctuations occur in the oral cavity due to the ingestion of hot or cold food and drink. In addition, more localized temperature increases may occur due to the highly exothermic nature of the setting reaction for some dental materials. The dental pulp is very sensitive to temperature change and in the healthy tooth is surrounded by dentine and enamel, which are re-

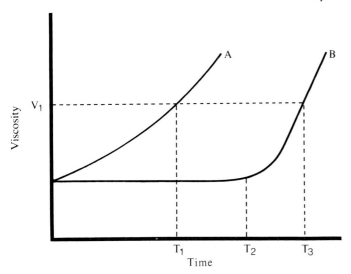

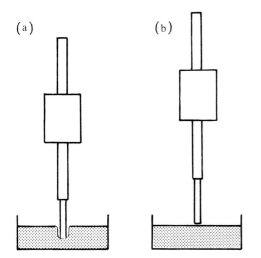

Fig. 2.19 Assessment of setting time by determination of resistance to penetration. (a) Material is unset. (b) Material is set.

latively good thermal insulators. It is important that materials which are used to restore teeth should not only offer a similar degree of insulation but also should not undergo a large temperature rise when setting *in situ*.

Another consequence of thermal change is dimensional change. Materials generally expand when heated and contract when cooled. These dimensional changes may cause serious problems for filling materials, particularly in the region of the tooth/restorative interface.

Thermal conductivity Thermal conductivity is defined as the rate of heat flow per unit temperature gradient. Thus, good conductors have high values of conductivity. Table 2.2 gives values of thermal conductivity for some dental materials along with those for enamel and dentine. It is clear that heat is conducted through metals and alloys more readily than through polymers such as acrylic resin. The relatively high value of conductivity for dental amalgam indicates that this material could not provide satisfactory insulation of the pulp. For this reason it is normal practice to use a cavity base of a cement such as zinc phosphate which has a lower thermal conductivity value.

Thermal conductivity is an equilibrium property and since most thermal stimuli encountered in the mouth are transitory in nature the value of *thermal diffusivity* may be of more practical use in predicting materials behaviour.

Thermal diffusivity Thermal diffusivity (D) is defined by the equation

$$D = \frac{K}{Cp \times \rho}$$

where K is the thermal conductivity, Cp is the heat capacity and ρ the density. This property gives a better indication of the way in which a material responds to transient thermal stimuli. Thus, if a cold drink is taken and the cooling effect on any tooth or restoration surface is maintained for only a second or two, the diffusivity allows calculation of the temperature change in the pulp. This should, naturally, be as small as possible.

Table 2.2 Thermal conductivity values of some selected dental materials

Material	Thermal conductivity W m^{-1} °C^{-1}
Enamel	0·92
Dentine	0·63
Acrylic resin	0·21
Dental amalgam	23·02
Zinc phosphate cement	1·17
Zinc oxide/eugenol cement	0·46
Silicate materials	0·75
Porcelain	1·05
Gold	291·70

Measurements of thermal diffusivity are often made by embedding a thermocouple in a specimen of material and plunging the specimen into a hot or cold liquid (Fig. 2.20a). If the temperature recorded by the thermocouple rapidly reaches that of the liquid, this indicates a high value of diffusivity. A slow response, on the other hand, indicates a lower value of diffusivity (Fig. 2.20b). In many circumstances a low value of diffusivity is preferred. However, there are occasions on which a high value is beneficial. For example, a denture base material, ideally, should have a high value of thermal diffusivity in order that the patient retains a satisfactory response to hot and cold stimuli in the mouth.

Exothermic reactions Many dental materials involve the mixing of two or more components followed by setting. The setting process often occurs *in situ* and very often the chemical reaction occurring during setting is exothermic in nature. For

Table 2.3 Temperature rise during setting of some selected materials (100 mg sample)

Material	Temperature rise °C
Zinc oxide/eugenol cement	0·2
Zinc phosphate cement	1·9
Acrylic resin	9·6
Composite resin	4·0
Glass ionomer cement	1·0

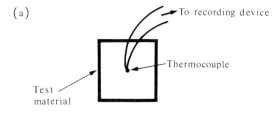

(a)

To recording device

Thermocouple

Test material

Fig. 2.20 Measuring thermal diffusivity by embedding a thermocouple in a sample of the material. The sample is plunged into a hot or cold fluid and temperature change plotted against time.

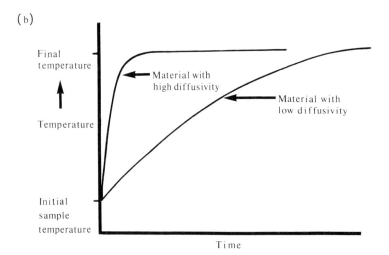

(b)

Final temperature

Material with high diffusivity

Material with low diffusivity

Temperature

Initial sample temperature

Time

industrial production processes, exothermic reactions must be closely controlled in order to avoid
explosions. For dental materials this is not a problem due to the relatively small sample sizes used.
However, the heat liberated and the associated rise
in temperature may cause clinical problems.

Table 2.3 gives typical values of temperature rise
recorded for small samples of some dental materials. Naturally, the temperature rise increases
with an increasing amount of material. Hence, due
regard must be paid to the possible effect that such
materials may have on the dental pulp when used
as restoratives, particularly when a large bulk of
material is used.

Coefficient of thermal expansion The linear coefficient of thermal expansion is defined as the fractional increase in length of a body for each degree
centigrade increase in temperature. Thus,

$$\alpha = \frac{\triangle L/L_0}{\triangle T} \, °C^{-1}$$

where the coefficient α is defined in terms of the
change in length $\triangle L$, the original length L_0 and the
temperature change $\triangle T$.

Because the values of α are often very small
numbers (typically $0.000025°C^{-1}$ for amalgam) they
are often quoted as parts per million (p.p.m.). For
example, the value for a typical amalgam specimen
would be quoted as 25 p.p.m. $°C^{-1}$. Values for
some common materials are given in Table 2.4.

This property is particularly important for filling
materials. When the patient takes a cold drink,
both the filling material and tooth substance contract, the amount of contraction depending on the
value of α for each. If the value of α for the
material is significantly greater than that for tooth
substance a small gap will develop down which
fluids containing bacteria can penetrate, as illustrated in Fig. 2.21. The magnitude of the gap,
shown as x in the diagram, is minimized for both hot
and cold stimuli if the values of α for tooth substance and filling are matched. Hence, it can be
seen from Table 2.4 that certain materials, for
example silicate cements, perform very well in this
respect, whilst others, such as acrylic resin, perform
badly.

In practice, however, the situation is not so clear
cut. Coefficient of thermal expansion is an equilibrium property and the expansion or contraction
due to transient stimuli is a function of both coefficient of thermal expansion and thermal diffusivity.

Table 2.4 Coefficient of thermal expansion values of
some selected materials

Material	Coefficient of thermal expansion (p.p.m. $°C^{-1}$)
Enamel	11.4
Dentine	8.0
Acrylic resin	90
Porcelain	4
Amalgam	25
Composite resins	25−60
Silicate cements	10

For filling materials, the most ideal combination of
properties would be a low value of diffusivity combined with a coefficient of thermal expansion value
similar to that for tooth substance.

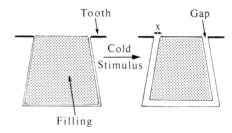

Fig. 2.21 Diagram illustrating the production of a marginal gap due to thermal contraction.

2.5 Adhesion

The property of adhesion is recognized as being of
major importance for filling materials, luting
materials and fissure sealants. In each case the aim
is to produce a tight seal between tooth substance
and material with minimal destruction of tooth
tissue.

Materials which are capable of 'bonding' two
surfaces together are called *adhesives* whilst the
material to which the adhesive is applied is termed
the *adherend*. In dentistry, an adhesive may,
typically, be required to 'bond' dentine and gold
or, if the adhesive also acts as a filling material,
may simply be required to attach to one surface,
for example enamel.

Bonding may be achieved by one of two mechanisms — *mechanical attachment* or *chemical
adhesion*.

In *mechanical attachment* the adhesive simply
engages in undercuts in the adherend surface as
shown in Fig. 2.22. When the surface irregularities
responsible for bonding have dimensions of only a

(a)

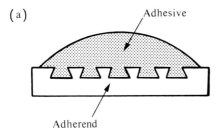

(b)

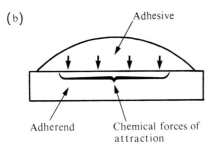

Fig. 2.22 Diagram illustrating the difference between (a) micromechanical attachment and (b) chemical adhesion.

few micrometres the process is known as *micromechanical attachment*. This should be distinguished from *macromechanical attachment* which forms the basis of retention for many filling materials, using undercut cavities. In the case of *chemical adhesion* the adhesive has a chemical affinity for the adherend surface. If the attraction is

caused by Van der Waals forces or hydrogen bonds, the resultant 'bond' may be relatively weak. On the other hand, the formation of ionic or covalent links may result in a stronger 'bond'.

Whichever mechanism of bonding is utilized the adhesive must be capable of *wetting* the adherend surface. In the case of mechanical attachment the adhesive must flow readily across the adherend surface and enter into all the surface undercuts in order to form the 'bond'. For chemical adhesion the adhesive must *wet* the adherend surface in order that intimate contact between the adhesive and adherend may result in the formation of specific links which cause 'bonding'.

The ability of an adhesive to wet an adherend surface is evaluated by measuring the *contact angle* which is formed when a drop of adhesive is applied to the surface. Fig. 2.23 shows that for good wetting, a low contact angle, ideally approaching $0°$, is required. High contact angles indicate poor wetting and globule formation, and would probably result in poor adhesion.

The main factors which affect the contact angle are the *surface tension* (ST) of the adhesive and the *surface free energy* (SFE) of the adherend. The condition which must prevail if low contact angles are to be achieved is:

$$SFE > ST$$

Hence, the surface free energy of the adherend must be maximized for best results.

The adherend surfaces most often concerned when dealing with dental adhesives are enamel and

(a)

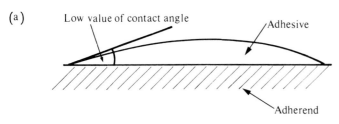

(b)

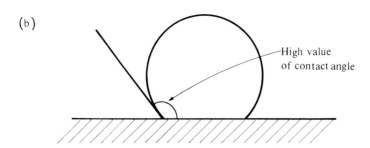

Fig. 2.23 Diagram showing (a) good wetting of an adherend surface and (b) poor wetting and globule formation.

dentine and the value of SFE for these surfaces is maximized by ensuring a clean, dry, oil-free surface at the time when the adhesive is applied.

2.6 Miscellaneous physical properties
Properties of materials which may influence their acceptability but which do not fall into any of the other categories are (1) dimensional changes during and after setting, (2) density and (3) colour.

Dimensional changes Dimensional accuracy is an important requirement of many dental materials. The success of many restorative procedures depends on dimensional changes which occur during impression recording, casting of alloys or setting of direct restorative materials.

The manipulation of many materials involves the mixing of two or more components followed by a chemical reaction which brings about setting. Chemical reactions are invariably accompanied by dimensional changes. In the case of polymerization reactions, a contraction normally occurs whereas other types of reaction may result in an expansion.

Where several stages are involved in the production of a restoration or appliance it is possible that dimensional changes occur at each stage. In such a case it is possible that an expansion at one stage can be used to partly counteract a contraction which occurs at another stage. For example, when constructing a cast metal restoration the setting expansion of the investment material partially compensates for the casting shrinkage of the alloy.

Dimensional changes may continue to occur in materials long after the apparent setting. There are many possible causes. Firstly, the changes may be due to continued slow setting or release of stresses set up during setting. Alternatively, they may be due to water absorption by, or loss of constituents from, the material. The degree to which the dimensions of a material alter after setting is said to be a measure of its *dimensional stability*.

Density Density is a fundamental property which affects design aspects of dental appliances. If, for example, one were choosing an alloy with which to construct components of an upper denture, it would be necessary to consider density. A bulky design in a heavy alloy would result in large displacing forces making retention difficult. In order to reduce

such destabilizing forces one may choose to use a lower density alloy and to keep the alloy bulk to a minimum.

Colour One of the most demanding requirements of dental restorative materials is that they should match the natural hard and soft tissues in appearance. Colour may be described quantitatively in terms of a three-dimensional colour chart such as that shown in Fig. 2.24. The three independent parameters represented in the diagram are:

(1) The dominant wavelength or *hue*, represented by the position on the circumference,

(2) The colour intensity or *chroma*, represented by the radial distance from the centre of the circle,

(3) The *brightness* as represented by the position in the vertical column.

The *hue* and *chroma* are inherent properties of materials whereas the *brightness* may be affected by factors such as surface finish.

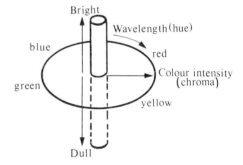

Fig. 2.24 Three-dimensional representation of colour, including wavelength of light, intensity and brightness.

2.7 Chemical properties
One of the main factors which determines the durability of a material used in the mouth is its chemical stability. Materials should not dissolve, erode or corrode, nor should they leach important constituents into the oral fluids.

Solubility and erosion The solubility of a material is simply a measurement of the extent to which it will dissolve in a given fluid, for example, water or saliva. Erosion, on the other hand, is a process which combines the chemical process of dissolution with a mild mechanical action. Hence it is possible to envisage a situation in which the surface layer of a material becomes weakened and undermined by

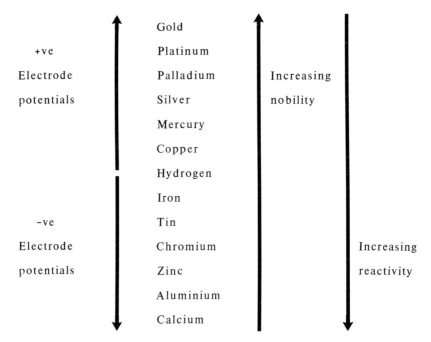

Fig. 2.25 Ranking orders of electrode potentials and reactivities for various metals.

dissolution and then becomes totally detached by mild abrasion.

These properties are particularly important for all restorative materials since a high solubility or poor resistance to erosion will severely limit the effective lifetime of the restoration.

When assessing the solubility or erosion rate of materials it is important to consider the vast range of conditions which may exist in the mouth. The pH of oral fluids may vary from pH 4 to pH 8·5, representing a range from mildly acidic to mildly alkaline. Highly acidic soft drinks and the use of chalk-containing toothpastes extend this range from a lower end of pH 2 up to pH 11. It is possible for a material to be stable at near neutral pH values but to erode rapidly at extremes of either acidity or alkalinity. This partially explains why certain materials perform adequately with some patients but not with others.

Standard tests of solubility often involve the storage of disc specimens of materials in water for a period of time, the result being quoted as the percentage weight loss of the disc. Such methods, however, often give misleading results. When comparing silicate and phosphate cements, for example, silicate materials appear more soluble in simple laboratory tests but in practice they are more durable than the phosphates.

Leaching of constituents Many materials, when placed in an aqueous environment, absorb water by a diffusion process. Constituents of the material may be lost into the oral fluids by a diffusion process commonly referred to as leaching. This may have serious consequences if it results in a change of material properties or if the leached material is toxic or irritant.

Some soft acrylic polymers used for cushioning the fitting surfaces of dentures rely on the presence of relatively large quantities of plasticizer in the acrylic resin for their softness. The slow leaching of plasticizer causes the resin to become hard and therefore ineffective as a cushion.

Occasionally leaching is used to the benefit of the patient. For example, in some cements containing calcium hydroxide, slow leaching causes an alkaline environment in the base of deep cavities. This has the dual benefit of being antibacterial and of encouraging secondary dentine formation.

Corrosion Corrosion is a term which specifically characterizes the chemical reactivity of metals and alloys. The major requirement of any such material used in the mouth is that it should have good corrosion resistance.

Metals and alloys are good electrical conductors

and many corrosion processes involve the setting up of an electrolytic cell as a first stage in the process.

The tendency of a metal to corrode can be predicted from its electrode potential. It can be seen from Fig. 2.25 that materials with large negative electrode potential values are more reactive whilst those with large positive values are far less reactive and are often referred to as *noble* metals. The electrode potential is a measure of the extent to which the reaction

$$M \rightarrow M^+ + \text{electron}$$

will occur.

In an electrolytic cell involving two metals, material is lost from the metal with the most negative electrode potential. Thus, when zinc and copper come into contact in the presence of a suitable electrolyte (Fig. 2.26), material loss occurs from the zinc by the reaction:

$$Zn \rightarrow Zn^{2+} + 2 \text{ electrons}$$

Hydrogen is liberated at the copper by the reaction:

$$2H^+ + 2 \text{ electrons} \rightarrow H_2$$

In this simple type of electrolytic cell the zinc is referred to as the *anode*. This is the electrode at which positive ions are formed and therefore the electrode at which corrosion occurs. The copper is referred to as the *cathode*. The more negative a value of electrode potential which a metal possesses the more likely it is to form the anode in an electrolytic cell.

If a voltmeter is placed between the anode and cathode an electrical potential difference can be measured, thus illustrating the flow of electrons within the electrolytic cell.

The conditions under which an electrolytic cell may be set up in the mouth involve the presence of two or more metals of different electrode potential and a suitable electrolyte. Saliva and tissue fluids are good electrolytes. The two metals may be derived from restorations constructed from different metals or alloys, or from areas of different composition within one restoration, for example amalgam, as illustrated in Fig. 2.27.

Generally, the more homogeneous the distribution of metal atoms within an alloy the less tendency there is for corrosion to occur. Consequently, many manufacturers of alloys carry out homogenization heat treatments to help to eliminate the possibility of electrolytic corrosion.

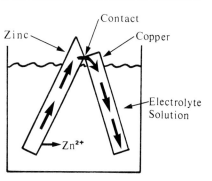

Fig. 2.26 Electrolytic cell involving two dissimilar metals in contact and an electrolyte. Corrosion of the most electronegative metal occurs.

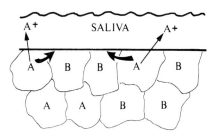

Fig. 2.27 An electrolytic cell involving different phases within one alloy. Saliva acts as the electrolyte. Phase A is more electronegative than phase B.

It can be seen from Fig. 2.25 that chromium has a negative value of electrode potential and is at the reactive end of the series of metals shown. It is therefore surprising to learn that chromium is included as a component of many alloys in order to improve corrosion resistance. This apparent contradiction can be explained by the *passivating effect*. Although chromium is electrochemically active it reacts readily forming a layer of chromic oxide which protects the metal or alloy from further decomposition.

Other factors which can affect the corrosion of metals and alloys are stress and surface roughness. Stress in metal components of appliances produced, for example, by excessive or continued bending can accelerate the rate of corrosion and may lead to failure by *stress corrosion cracking*. Pits in rough surfaces can lead to the setting up of small corrosion cells in which the material at the bottom of the pit acts as the anode and that at the surface acts as the cathode. The mechanism of this type of corrosion, sometimes referred to as *concentration cell corrosion*, is complicated but is caused by the fact that pits tend to become filled with debris which reduces the oxygen concentration in the base of the pit compared with the surface. In order to reduce corrosion by this mechanism, metals and alloys used in the mouth should be polished to remove surface irregularities.

2.8 Biological properties

It is a primary requirement of any dental material that it should be harmless to the patient and to those involved in its manufacture and handling. Whilst the manufacture of materials may involve the use of relatively toxic raw materials, close control of production processes reduces or eliminates the risk to personnel.

Ideally, a material placed into a patient's mouth should be non-toxic, non-irritant, have no carcinogenic or allergic potential and, if used as a filling material, should be harmless to the pulp.

Biological evaluation of dental materials is carried out on three levels. At the first level, simple screening tests can be used to evaluate acute systemic toxicity, irritational potential and carcinogenic potential. The second level of testing involves limited usage tests in experimental animals. For example, when evaluating filling materials it is common to place restorations in the teeth of monkeys or ferrets. If the tests carried out at the first and second levels produce satisfactory results then it is possible to consider moving to the third level of testing — the controlled clinical trial involving volunteer human subjects. Hence, every effort is made to ensure the safety of new products.

The effect of materials on the dentists, surgery assistants and technicians involved in their handling is an important consideration. Materials are normally in their most reactive and potentially harmful state during mixing and manipulation. In addition, dental personnel may be exposed to materials over a long period of time. For example, mercury is known to have certain toxic effects and the most potent mechanism for incorporation of mercury into the body is by inhaling mercury vapour. A patient may spend only a few minutes each year in a mercury-contaminated dental surgery and is thus subjected to only minimal exposure. The dentist and his assistant, on the other hand, may spend all of their working lives in such an environment. The need for adequate mercury hygiene is therefore apparent.

Materials used for certain applications have specific biological requirements which will be discussed in the relevant chapters dealing with those groups of products.

3

Gypsum Products for Models and Dies

3.1 Introduction

Gypsum is a naturally occurring, white powdery mineral with the chemical name calcium sulphate dihydrate ($CaSO_4 \cdot 2H_2O$). Gypsum products used in dentistry are based on calcium sulphate hemihydrate ($(CaSO_4)_2 \cdot H_2O$). Their main uses are for models, dies and investments, the latter being considered in Chap. 5.

Many dental restorations and appliances are constructed outside the patient's mouth using models and dies which should be accurate replicas of the patient's hard and soft tissues.

The term *model* is normally used when referring to a replica of several teeth and their associated soft tissues or, alternatively, to an edentulous arch. The term *die* is normally used when referring to a replica of a single tooth.

The morphology of the hard and soft tissues is recorded in an impression and models and dies are prepared using materials which are initially fluid and can be poured into the impression, then harden to form a rigid replica.

Many materials have been used for producing models and dies but the most popular are the materials based on gypsum products.

3.2 Requirements of model and die materials

The main requirements of model and die materials are dimensional accuracy and adequate mechanical properties. The accuracy of fit of any restoration or appliance constructed outside the mouth depends *inter alia* on the dimensional accuracy of the replica on which it is constructed. Thus, the dimensional changes which occur during and after the setting of these model materials should, ideally, be minimal in order to produce an accurate model or die. The final 'fit' of the appliance may depend upon a balancing of small expansions or contractions which occur at different stages in its construction and it would be unwise to consider, in isolation, dimen-

sional changes occurring with the model and die materials.

Although small dimensional changes during setting can often be tolerated and even compensated for, changes occurring during storage are a more serious problem. Hence, the dimensional stability after setting should be as good as possible.

The material should, ideally, be fluid at the time it is poured into the impression so that fine detail can be recorded. A low contact angle between the model and impression materials would help to minimize the presence of surface voids on the set model by encouraging surface wetting.

The set material should be sufficiently strong to resist accidental fracture and hard enough to resist abrasion during the carving of a wax pattern.

The material should be compatible with all the other materials with which it comes into contact. For example, the set model should easily be removed from the impression without damage to its surface and fracture of teeth. It should give a good colour contrast with the various waxes which are often used to produce wax patterns.

3.3 Composition

Gypsum products used in dentistry are formed by driving off part of the water of crystallization from gypsum to form calcium sulphate hemihydrate.

$$\text{Gypsum} \rightarrow \text{Gypsum product} + \text{Water}$$
$$2CaSO_4 \cdot 2H_2O \rightarrow (CaSO_4)_2 \cdot H_2O + 3H_2O$$

Calcium	Calcium
sulphate	sulphate
dihydrate	hemihydrate

Applications of gypsum products in dentistry involve the reverse of the above reaction. The hemihydrate is mixed with water and reacts to form the dihydrate.

$$(CaSO_4)_2 \cdot H_2O + 3H_2O \rightarrow 2CaSO_4 \cdot 2H_2O$$

The various types of gypsum product used in dentistry are chemically identical, in that they con-

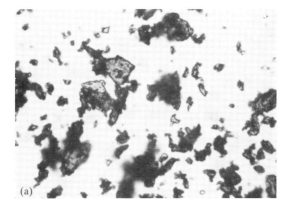

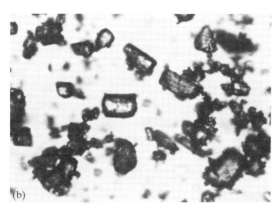

Fig. 3.1 (a) Particles of calcium sulphate β-hemihydrate (dental plaster) (× 240). (b) Particles of calcium sulphate α-hemihydrate (dental stone) (× 240).

sist of calcium sulphate hemihydrate, but they may differ in physical form depending upon the method used for their manufacture.

Dental plaster (*plaster of Paris*) Dental plaster is produced by a process known as calcination. Gypsum is heated to a temperature of about 120°C in order to drive off part of the water of crystallization. This produces irregular, porous particles which are sometimes referred to as β-hemihydrate particles (Fig. 3.1a).

Dental stone Dental stones may be produced by one of two methods. If gypsum is heated to about 125°C under steam pressure in an autoclave a more regular and less porous hemihydrate is formed (Fig. 3.1b). This is sometimes referred to as an α-hemihydrate.

Alternatively, gypsum may be boiled in a solution of a salt such as $CaCl_2$. This gives a material

Table 3.1 Water/powder ratios for gypsum model and die materials

	Water (ml)	Powder (g)	W/P ratio (ml/g)
Plaster	50−60	100	0·55
Stone	20−35	100	0·30
Theoretical ratio	18·6*	100	0·186

*Sometimes referred to as gauging water.

similar to that produced by autoclaving but with even less porosity. Manufacturers normally add small quantities of a dye to dental stones in order that they may be differentiated from dental plaster, which is white.

3.4 Manipulation and setting characteristics

Plaster and stone powders are mixed with water to produce a workable mix. Hydration of the hemihydrate then occurs producing the gypsum model or die.

Table 3.1 gives an indication of the water/powder ratio used for each material along with the theoretical ratio required to satisfy the chemical reaction which occurs. Although a ratio of only 0·186 is required to satisfy the reaction, such a mix would be too dry and unworkable. In the case of the more dense material, dental stone, a ratio of about 0·3 is required to produce a workable mix, whereas for the more porous plaster a higher W/P ratio of 0·55 is required. The excess water is absorbed by the porosities of the plaster particles. Considerable quantities of air may be incorporated during mixing and this may lead to porosity within the set material. Air porosity may be reduced by vibrating the mix of plaster or stone in order to bring air bubbles to the surface.

The setting process begins rapidly after mixing the powder and water. The first stage in the process is that the water becomes saturated with hemihydrate, which has a solubility of around 0·8 percent at room temperature. The dissolved hemihydrate is then rapidly converted to dihydrate which has a much lower solubility of around 0·2 percent. Since the solubility limit of the dihydrate is immediately exceeded it begins to crystallize out of solution. The process continues until most of the hemihydrate is converted to dihydrate.

The crystals of dihydrate are spherulitic in nature and grow from specific sites called nuclei of crystal-

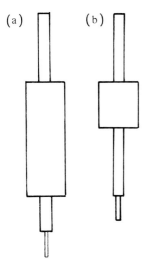

(a)   (b)

Fig. 3.2 Indentors used to assess setting characteristics of gypsum products. Sometimes referred to as Gilmore needles. Ability to support needle (b) indicates the initial set. Ability to support needle (a) indicates 'final' set.

lization. These may be small particles of impurity, such as unconverted gypsum crystals, within the hemihydrate powder.

The material should be used as soon as possible after mixing since its viscosity increases to the stage where the material is unworkable within a few minutes. Two stages can be identified during setting. The first is the time at which the material develops the properties of a weak solid and will not flow readily. At this time, often referred to as the initial setting time, it is possible to carve away excess material with a knife. The materials continue to develop strength for some time after initial setting and eventually reach a stage when the models or dies are strong and hard enough to be worked upon. The time taken to reach this stage is referred to as the final setting time, although this term is misleading since it implies that the material has reached its ultimate strength. This may not be reached until several hours after mixing.

The setting characteristics of gypsum products are often measured in terms of their ability to resist penetration by needles, such as those shown in Fig. 3.2. The heavier needle has a smaller tip diameter than the lighter one and hence applies a considerably greater pressure to the surface of the material under test. The initial setting time is defined as the time taken for the material to develop sufficient strength such that it is able to support the lighter of the needles. The time at which the material is able to support the heavier needle has doubtful practical significance since it indicates a time somewhere between the initial and final setting times and is not indicative of the fact that the model or die is hard enough to be used.

The setting reaction is exothermic, the maximum temperature being reached during the stage when final hardening occurs (Fig. 3.3). It is interesting to note that the temperature rise is still negligible at the time of the initial set.

Another physical change which accompanies setting is a small expansion caused by the outward thrust of growing crystals as shown in Fig. 3.4. The

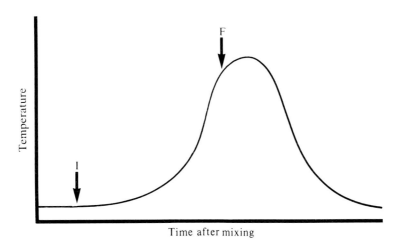

Fig. 3.3 Temperature–time profile for a gypsum material during setting. Points I and F correspond to the initial set and final set points indicated by indentors (Fig. 3.2).

(a)

(b)

(c)

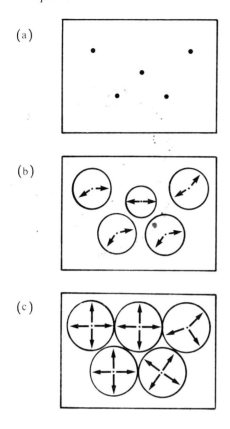

Fig. 3.4 Diagram showing growth of spherulitic gypsum crystals, indicating (a) the nuclei from which crystals grow, (b) spherulitic growth and (c) the outward thrust as spherulites make contact.

maximum rate of expansion occurs at the time when the temperature is increasing most rapidly. The expansion is, in fact, only apparent since the set material contains a considerable volume of porosity. If the material is placed in water at the initial set stage, considerably more expansion occurs during setting. This increased expansion is called *hygroscopic expansion* and is sometimes used to increase the setting expansion of gypsum-bonded investment materials (Chap. 5).

Conrol of setting time Factors which control the setting times of gypsum products can be divided into those controlled by manufacturers and those controlled by the operator.

The manufacturer can control the concentration of nucleating agents in the hemihydrate powder. A higher concentration of nucleating agent, produced by ageing or from unconverted calcium sulphate dihydrate, results in more rapid crystallization. Also, the manufacturers may add chemical accelerators or retarders. Potassium sulphate is a commonly used accelerator which is thought to act by increasing the solubility of the hemihydrate. Borax is the most widely used retarder, although the mechanism by which it works is not clear.

Factors under the control of the operator are temperature, water/powder ratio and mixing time. Surprisingly, temperature variation has little effect on the setting times of gypsum products. This is due to the fact that the setting involves a dissolution of one sparingly soluble salt followed by crystallization of another. Increasing the temperature accelerates the solution process but retards the crystallization. Thus the two effects tend to cancel out. Increasing the water/powder ratio retards setting by decreasing the concentration of crystallization nuclei. Increasing mixing time has the opposite effect. This accelerates setting by breaking up dihydrate crystals during the early stages of setting, thus producing more nuclei on which crystallization can be initiated. These effects are shown in Fig. 3.5.

Control of setting expansion In order to produce an accurate model or die it is necessary to maintain the setting expansion at as low a value as possible. Accelerators or retarders which are added by manufacturers in order to control the setting time also have the effect of reducing the setting expansion and are sometimes referred to as *anti-expansion agents*. The final values of expansion observed for typical materials are 0·4 percent for plaster and 0·1 percent for stone. The very low value of expansion for stone may be considered negligible in terms of its effect on the accuracy of restorations or appliances which are to be constructed.

Alterations in water/powder ratio and mixing time have only a minimal effect on setting expansion.

3.5 **Properties of the set material**
The strength of gypsum depends, primarily, on the porosity of the set material and the time for which the material is allowed to dry out after setting.

The porosity, and hence the strength, is proportional to the water/powder ratio as shown in Fig. 3.6.

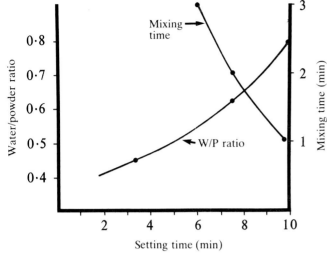

Fig. 3.5 The effect of water/powder ratio and mixing time on setting time for a typical dental plaster.

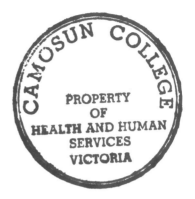

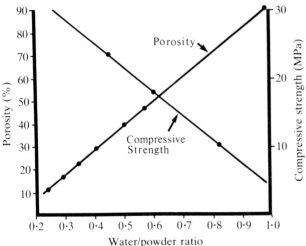

Fig. 3.6 The effect of water/powder ratio on the porosity and compressive strength of gypsum products.

Since stone is always mixed at a lower water/powder ratio than plaster it is less porous and consequently much stronger and harder.

Although a gypsum model or die may appear completely set within a relatively short period its strength increases significantly if it is allowed to stand for a few hours. The increase in strength is a function of the loss of excess water by evaporation. It is thought that evaporation of water causes a precipitation of any dissolved dihydrate and that this effectively cements together the crystals of gypsum formed during setting.

Despite precautions which may be taken to ensure optimum mechanical properties, gypsum is a very brittle material. It is relatively rigid but has a poor impact strength and is likely to fracture if dropped. Attempts to improve the mechanical pro-

perties have involved the impregnation by a polymer such as acrylic resin and the use of wetting agents which enable the materials to be used at a lower water/powder ratio.

The dimensional stability of gypsum is good. Following setting, further changes in dimensions are immeasurable and the materials are sufficiently rigid to resist deformations when work is being carried out upon them.

3.6 Applications
When strength, hardness and accuracy are required dental stones are normally used in preference to dental plaster. The stone materials are less likely to be damaged during the laying down and carving of

a wax pattern and give optimal dimensional accuracy. Thus, these materials are used when any work is to be carried out on the model or die as would be the case when constructing a denture on a model or a cast alloy crown on a die.

When mechanical properties and accuracy are not of primary importance the cheaper dental plaster is used. Thus, plaster is often used for mounting stone models onto articulators and for preparing study models.

3.7 Advantages and disadvantages
Gypsum model and die materials have the advantages of being inexpensive and easy to use. The accuracy and dimensional stability are good and they are able to reproduce fine detail from the impression, providing precautions are taken to prevent blow holes.

The mechanical properties are not ideal and the brittle nature of gypsum occasionally leads to fracture — particularly through the teeth, which form the weakest part of any model.

Problems occasionally arise when gypsum model and die materials are used in conjunction with alginate impressions. The surface of the model may remain relatively soft due to the retarding effect of borax which is present in many alginate materials. Despite these observations it cannot be said that gypsum products are incompatible with alginate impression materials since problems arise very infrequently.

Alternative materials for the production of models and dies exist but are hardly ever used. These include various resins, cements and dental amalgam. The alternatives may be stronger but are generally less stable, difficult to use and more expensive. The surface of a gypsum die can be hardened by electroplating the impression prior to constructing the die. The thin layer of metal, copper for impression compound and silver for some elastomers, is transferred to the surface of the die on separation from the impression.

4 $\qquad$ Waxes

4.1 Introduction
Waxes form a group of thermoplastic materials which are normally solids at room temperature but melt, without decomposition, to form mobile liquids. They are, essentially, soft substances with poor mechanical properties and their primary uses in dentistry are to form *patterns* of appliances prior to casting.

Following the production of a stone model or die (Chap. 3), the next stage in the formation of many dental appliances, dentures or restorations is the production of a wax pattern of the appliance on the model. The wax pattern defines the shape and size of the resulting appliance and is eventually replaced by either a polymer or an alloy using the *lost-wax technique*. Methods which involve the production of a model followed by the laying down of a wax pattern are known as *indirect techniques*. Some dental restorations, such as inlays, may be produced by a *direct wax pattern* technique in which the inlay wax is adapted and shaped in the prepared cavity in the mouth. Waxes used in the production of patterns by either the direct or indirect technique must have very precisely controlled properties in order that well-fitting restorations or appliances may be constructed. Other waxes used in dentistry have less rigorous property requirements. One such material is used by manufacturers for attaching denture teeth to display sheets (*carding wax*). Another product is used for boxing in impressions prior to making a gypsum model (*boxing-in wax*). A third material is used for temporarily joining two components of an appliance, for example, during soldering (*sticky wax*).

An important group of waxes used in dentistry are the impression waxes. These are discussed on p.109.

4.2 Requirements of wax-pattern materials
The major requirements of waxes used to construct wax patterns by either the direct or indirect technique are:

(1) The wax pattern must conform to the exact size, shape and contour of the appliance which is to be constructed,

(2) No dimensional change should take place in the wax pattern once it has been formed,

(3) After formation of the casting mould, it should be possible to remove the wax by boiling out or burning without leaving a residue.

The ability to record detail depends on the flow of the material at the moulding temperature, which is just above mouth temperature for direct techniques and just above room temperature for indirect techniques. Accuracy and dimensional stability depend on dimensional changes which occur during solidification and cooling of the wax. Distortions may also occur if thermal stresses are introduced.

4.3 Composition of waxes
Dental waxes are composed of mixtures of thermoplastic materials which can be softened by heating then hardened by cooling. The major components may be of mineral, animal or vegetable origin.

Mineral Paraffin wax and the closely related microcrystalline wax are both obtained from petroleum residues following distillation. They are both hydrocarbons, paraffin wax being a simple straight-chain hydrocarbon whilst the microcrystalline material has a branched structure as shown in Fig. 4.1.

Paraffin waxes soften in the temperature range 37–55°C and melt in the range 48–70°C. They are brittle at room temperature. Microcrystalline waxes melt in the range 65–90°C and when added to paraffin waxes they raise its melting point. At the same time they lower the softening temperature and render the material less brittle than paraffin wax alone.

Animal Beeswax, derived from honeycombs, con-

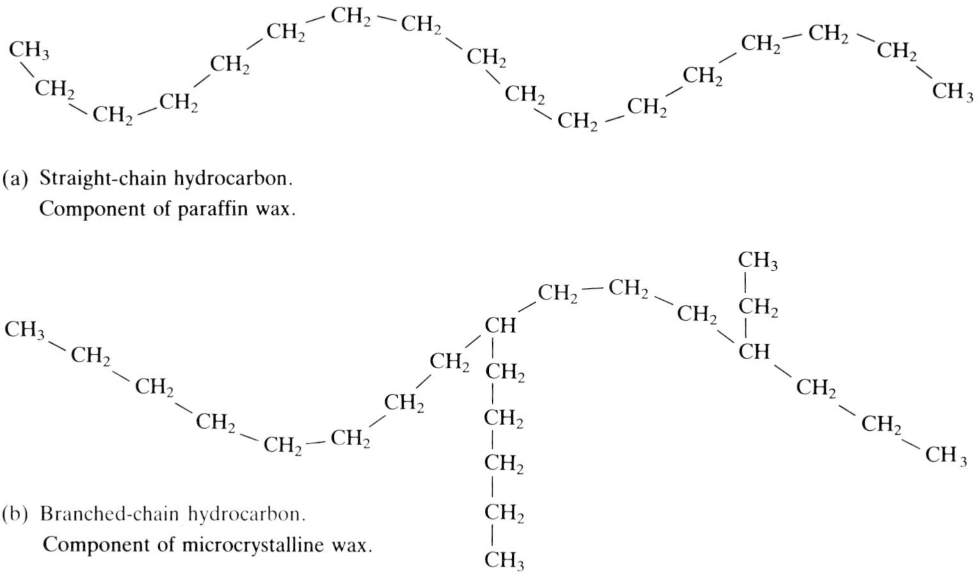

(a) Straight-chain hydrocarbon.
    Component of paraffin wax.

(b) Branched-chain hydrocarbon.
    Component of microcrystalline wax.

Fig. 4.1 Structures of hydrocarbons found in some waxes.

sists of a partially crystalline natural polyester and is often blended with paraffin wax in order to modify the properties of the latter. The effect of adding beeswax to paraffin wax is to render the material less brittle and to reduce the extent to which it will flow under stress at temperatures just below the melting point.

Vegetable Carnauba wax and candelilla wax are derived from trees and plants. They are blended with paraffin wax in order to control the softening temperature and modify properties.

4.4 Properties of dental waxes

Waxes are generally characterized by their thermal properties such as *melting point* and *solid–solid transition temperature* which is closely related to the *softening temperature* observed in practice. The *coefficient of thermal expansion* is a major factor affecting accuracy. *Dimensional stability* is primarily a function of the magnitude of the stresses which become incorporated during thermal contraction after moulding. Important mechanical properties are *brittleness* and the degree of *flow* which a material will undergo in its working temperature range.

Thermal properties All the waxes used in dentistry have a predominantly crystalline structure and are characterized by a well-defined melting point. Inspection of a typical thermograph (Fig. 4.2) shows that a second endothermic peak exists at a temperature somewhat lower than the melting point. This peak is indicative of a solid–solid transition involving a change in the crystal structure of the wax. The change in crystal structure is accompanied by a change in mechanical properties and the wax is converted from a relatively brittle solid to a much softer, mouldable material. For this reason, the solid–solid transition temperature is sometimes referred to as the *softening temperature*. For many applications of waxes the softening temperature should be just above mouth temperature. This is in order that the material may be introduced into the mouth in a mouldable state but will become relatively rigid at mouth temperature. The manufacturers can control the melting point and softening temperature by blending mixtures of various mineral, animal and vegetable components.

Waxes are very poor thermal conductors and must be maintained above the solid–solid transition temperature for long enough to allow thorough softening to occur throughout the material before moulding is attempted.

Following moulding, the waxes are allowed to cool. During this cooling period they may undergo potentially significant contraction due to the high values of coefficient of expansion exhibited by

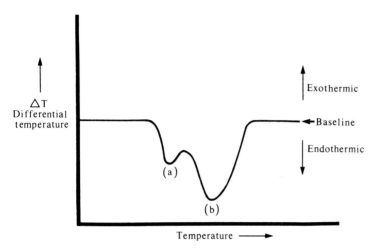

these products.

The thermal contraction may not be fully exhibited immediately after cooling. The low thermal conductivity values of the materials result in solidification of the surface layers of the wax well before the bulk becomes rigid. This reduces the magnitude of the thermal contraction and produces significant internal stresses. Dimensional changes may occur due to relief of the stresses. This is more likely to occur at elevated temperatures. Greater stresses may be incorporated if the wax is not properly softened before moulding.

The usual method for softening wax is to use a bunsen burner. In order to achieve even heating it is important that the wax should be held in the warm rising air above the flame and not in the flame itself. If the surface becomes shiny it indicates that the wax is becoming too hot and the outer layers are beginning to melt.

Heating in warm water causes more regular softening although this method has been frowned upon since it was thought that some constituents may be leached out and small quantities of water may become incorporated causing an alteration in properties. These problems are probably overstated since most waxes contain few leachable components.

The ideal method for softening wax is to use a wax 'annealer'. This is a thermostatically controlled oven which keeps the wax at a constant temperature, just above the softening point, ready for use. The 'annealer' is most useful for inlay waxes.

Mechanical properties A major factor which determines the mouldability and stability of a wax is its *flow* value. This property is related to *creep* which

is discussed on p.16. Creep and flow are both measured by applying a load to a cylindrical specimen and measuring the extent to which the specimen becomes compressed after a given time. Materials should, ideally, exhibit considerable flow at the moulding temperature but should show little or no flow at mouth temperature or room temperature so that they are not easily distorted.

Brittleness is another important property which the manufacturers can, to some extent, control. For some waxes, for example denture waxes, toughness is required since the wax denture base may have to be removed from a slightly undercut cast many times without fracturing. In other cases, such as inlay waxes, brittleness is preferred in order that the wax will fracture rather than distort on removal from an undercut cavity. This will indicate to the dental surgeon that a modification to the cavity shape is required.

4.5 **Applications**
Apart from their uses as impression materials, the major applications of waxes in dentistry are as modelling waxes and inlay waxes, collectively termed pattern waxes.

Modelling waxes The manufacture of dentures involves several stages with wax being used in at least two of these.

Following the production of a stone model from an impression, a wax 'rim' is constructed, either directly on the model, or on a denture base which has been adapted to the model. The rim is inserted into the patient's mouth at the 'registration' stage in order to ensure a satisfactory occlusal relationship. The next stage is to mount artificial teeth on the wax rim and to check the suitability of the wax denture at the 'try in' stage.

Waxes used for this purpose should have a softening temperature well above mouth temperature so that they are not distorted at either the 'registration' or 'try in' stages. They should be tough in order to reduce the chances of fracture during removal from the stone model.

Modelling waxes consist mainly of mixtures of paraffin wax and beeswax and have melting points in the range 49–58°C. They are generally supplied in sheet form, the sheets being produced either by rolling or by cutting from a block. Rolled sheets often change shape on softening due to the relief of stresses which are introduced during rolling.

Although the softening temperatures of modelling waxes are above mouth temperature the materials will slightly soften and distort if left in the mouth for more than a few minutes. This should be taken into account during registration and try in.

Modelling waxes are tough enough to resist fracture when withdrawn from shallow undercuts. When the wax denture is invested, prior to formation of an acrylic denture base, the wax can be removed from the mould by melting in boiling water, leaving no detectable residue.

Some metal components of partial dentures are formed in wax on the model. Small sheets of casting wax are used, which have been rolled to a precise thickness, according to the metal gauge required. In manipulating this wax it is important that the thickness is maintained. It is usual to soften it in hot water and adapt it into position with a soft material such as cotton wool or rubber.

Denture base-plate materials Denture modelling waxes may soften and distort if left in the mouth for more than a few minutes, as mentioned in the previous section. For this reason, shellac, a wax-like resin which is more stable at mouth temperature, has been used for construction of the temporary denture base. The wax rim is then built on top of this more stable base. Shellac is a natural beetle exudate which has a considerably higher softening temperature than ordinary modelling wax. Care must be taken to ensure thorough softening prior to moulding, otherwise considerable stresses are introduced which eventually lead to distortion.

Another widely used approach to denture construction is to use either a temporary or permanent acrylic base-plate on which to construct the wax rim. The advantages and disadvantages of the various approaches are beyond the scope of this book and are covered adequately in other excellent texts.

Inlay waxes Wax patterns for inlays can be produced either by a direct or indirect technique as mentioned previously. The use of direct wax patterns is normally reserved only for the most simple, single-surface inlays involving no cuspal coverage. These patterns can be removed from the prepared cavity with a minimum of distortion.

For direct wax patterns the softened wax is forced into the tooth cavity and held under pressure until it cools. The wax should soften just above mouth temperature and should not be raised to a higher temperature than necessary, in order to reduce the magnitude of thermal contractions and internal stresses. In addition, the softening temperature must be tolerated without pain by the patient. Dimensional changes caused by stress relief are minimized by investing the pattern as soon as possible.

The material should be hard at mouth temperature and when removed from the cavity should fracture rather than flow if the cavity has unwanted undercuts. This enables the undercuts to be located and removed.

The wax should ideally have a good colour contrast with enamel and be easy to carve without flaking so that the exposed surfaces of wax can be easily carved to shape and the margins readily observed.

The required properties are produced by using a blend of several types of wax including paraffin wax, carnauba, candelilla and beeswax with small quantities of other resins.

The procedure for indirect patterns is similar to that described for direct patterns except that the softened wax is forced into a cavity on the gypsum die. Since this procedure is carried out at room temperature rather than mouth temperature, inlay waxes for indirect patterns may soften at a somewhat lower temperature than direct pattern waxes, although the softening temperature should not be so low that the wax will flow at room temperature. The value of thermal contraction for the indirect technique is much lower as a result of the lower softening temperature.

Waxes used in the direct technique are referred

to as type I inlay waxes and those used in the indirect technique are referred to as type II inlay waxes. The two types are not interchangeable and no attempt should be made to use a type I material in the indirect technique and vice versa.

5   Investments

5.1 Introduction

Following the production of a wax pattern by either the direct or indirect method (Chap. 4), the next stage in many dental procedures involves the *investment* of the pattern to form a mould. A sprue is attached to the pattern and the assemblage is located in a casting ring (Fig. 5.1). Investment material is poured around the wax pattern whilst still in a fluid state. When the investment sets hard, the wax and sprue former are removed by softening and/or burning out, to leave a mould which can be filled with an alloy using a casting technique.

In the case of acrylic denture production the base-plate wax is invested in a two-part split mould using dental plaster or stone as investment. Following removal of the wax the resulting mould is filled with acrylic resin.

5.2 Requirements of investments for alloy casting procedures

The investment material forms the mould into which an alloy will be cast and it therefore follows that the accuracy of the casting can be no better than the accuracy of the mould.

The investment should be capable of reproducing the shape, size and detail recorded in the wax pattern. Since casting is carried out at very high temperatures, often in excess of 1000°C, the investment mould should be capable of maintaining its shape and integrity at these elevated temperatures. In addition, the investment should have a sufficiently high value of compressive strength at the casting temperature so that it can withstand the stresses set up when the molten metal enters the mould.

Alloy castings undergo considerable contraction when cooling from the casting temperature to room temperature. Such contraction may result in a casting with a very poor fit, for example a simple class I inlay would be loose fitting, whereas a crown would be too small and short at the margin. One function of the investment mould is to compensate for this casting shrinkage. This is generally achieved by a combination of setting expansion during the hardening of the investment mould and thermal expansion during the heating of the mould to the casting temperature.

The main factors involved in the selection of investment material are the casting temperature to be used and the type of alloy to be cast. Some gold alloys are cast at relatively low casting temperatures of around 900°C whilst some chromium alloys require casting temperatures of around 1450°C.

The investment which is best able to retain its integrity at the casting temperature and able to provide the necessary compensation for casting shrinkage is chosen.

5.3 Available materials

Investment materials consist of a mixture of a refractory material, normally silica, which is capable of withstanding very high temperatures without degradation, and a binder which binds the refractory particles together. The nature of the binder characterizes the material.

There are three main groups of investment material in common use. They are referred to as

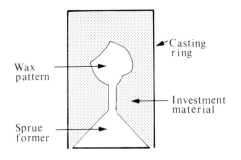

Fig. 5.1 Diagram illustrating how an investment mould is constructed from a wax pattern.

gypsum-bonded, silica-bonded or *phosphate-bonded.*

Gypsum-bonded materials

These materials are supplied as powders which are mixed with water and are composed of a mixture of silica (SiO_2) and calcium sulphate hemihydrate (gypsum product) together with other minor components including powdered graphite or powdered copper and various modifiers to control setting time.

Silica is a refractory material which adequately withstands the temperatures used during casting. It is available in three allotropic forms — quartz, cristobalite and tridymite — which are all chemically identical but differ slightly in crystalline form. Quartz and cristobalite are used extensively in investments. In addition to imparting the necessary refractory properties to the investment, the silica is responsible for producing much of the expansion which is necessary to compensate for the casting shrinkage of the alloy. The expansion is accomplished by a combination of simple thermal expansion coupled with a crystalline 'inversion' which results in a significant expansion. Quartz undergoes *inversion* at a temperature of 575°C from the so-called 'low' form or α-quartz to the so-called 'high' form or β-quartz. For cristobalite, conversion from the 'low' to the 'high' form occurs at a lower temperature of around 210°C. The expansion is probably due to a straightening of chemical bonds to form a less dense crystal structure as illustrated in Fig. 5.2. The change is reversible and both quartz and cristobalite revert back to the 'low' form on cooling. The overall thermal expansion and *inversion* expansion of materials containing cristobalite is greater than those containing quartz as illustrated in Fig. 5.3.

The calcium sulphate hemihydrate is an essential component since it reacts with water to form calcium sulphate dihydrate (gypsum) which effectively binds together the refractory silica. The chemistry of setting and important properties of gypsum products are dealt with in Chap. 3. The setting expansion of the calcium sulphate dihydrate, when mixed with water, is used to partially compensate for the shrinkage of the alloy which occurs on casting. Further compensation can be achieved by employing the hygroscopic setting expansion which occurs if the investment mould is placed into water at the initial set stage. The latter method is known as the *water immersion* hygroscopic expansion technique and can result in an expansion of five times the normal setting expansion. Another method is the *water added* technique in which a measured volume of water is placed on the upper surface of the investment material within the casting ring. This produces a more readily controlled expansion. Hygroscopic expansion is further encouraged by lining the casting ring with a layer of damp asbestos which is able to feed water to a large surface area of the investment mould. The latter technique is routinely employed even when no attempt is made to maximize hygroscopic expansion by immersing in water or adding water.

The mechanism of hygroscopic expansion is not fully understood. However, it may be envisaged that water is attracted between crystals by capillary action and that the extra separation of particles causes an expansion. The magnitude of the hygroscopic setting expansion which occurs with gypsum-bonded investments is greater than that which occurs with gypsum model and die materials.

Gypsum alone is not satisfactory as an investment for alloy casting since it contracts on heating as water is lost and fractures before reaching the casting temperature. The magnitude of the contraction, which occurs rapidly above 320°C, is significantly reduced in investment materials by the incorporation of sodium chloride and boric acid.

Silica-bonded materials

These materials consist of powdered quartz or

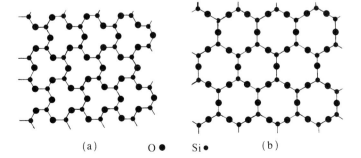

(a)   O ●   Si ●   (b)

Fig. 5.2 Bond straightening during 'inversion' of quartz at 575°C. (a) More dense structure existing below 575°C. (b) Less dense structure existing above 575°C.

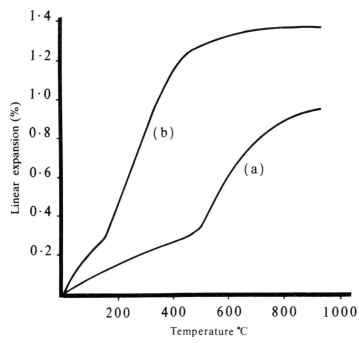

Fig. 5.3 Linear expansion versus temperature curves for two types of investment. (a) Containing quartz. (b) Containing cristobalite.

cristobalite which is bonded together with silica gel. On heating, the silica gel turns into silica so that the completed mould is a tightly packed mass of silica particles.

The binder solution is generally prepared by mixing ethyl silicate or one of its oligomers with a mixture of dilute hydrochloric acid and industrial spirit. The industrial spirit improves the mixing of ethyl silicate and water which are otherwise immissible. A slow hydrolysis of ethyl silicate occurs producing a sol of silicic acid with the liberation of ethyl alcohol as a byproduct.

$$(C_2H_5O)_4Si + 4H_2O \rightarrow Si(OH)_4 + 4C_2H_5OH$$

The silicic acid sol forms silica gel on mixing with quartz or cristobalite powder under alkaline conditions. The necessary pH is achieved by the presence of magnesium oxide in the powder.

Stock solutions of the hydrolysed ethyl silicate binder are normally made and stored in dark bottles. The solution gels slowly on standing and its viscosity may increase noticeably after three or four weeks. When this happens it is necessary to make up a fresh solution.

Simultaneous hydrolysis and gelation can be promoted by amines such as piperidine. Unfortunately, such a procedure is accompanied by an unacceptable shrinkage which is a result, mainly, of the hydrolysis reaction.

In order that the material should have sufficient strength at the casting temperature it is necessary to incorporate as much powder as possible into the binder solution. This process is aided by a gradation of particle sizes such that small grains fill in the spaces between the larger grains. A very thick, almost dry mix of investment is used and it is vibrated in order to encourage close packing and produce as strong an investment as possible.

A small shrinkage occurs during the early stages of the heating of the investment prior to casting. This is due to loss of water and alcohol from the gel. The contraction is followed by a more substantial thermal expansion and inversion expansion of the silica similar to that for gypsum-bonded investments.

Phosphate-bonded materials

These materials consist of a powder containing silica, magnesium oxide and ammonium phosphate. On mixing with water or a colloidal silica solution, a reaction between the phosphate and oxide occurs to form magnesium ammonium phosphate.

$$NH_4 \cdot H_2PO_4 + MgO + 5H_2O \rightarrow$$
$$Mg \cdot NH_4 \cdot PO_4 \cdot 6H_2O$$

This binds the silica together to form the set investment mould. The formation of the magnesium ammonium phosphate involves a hydration reaction followed by crystallization similar to that for the formation of gypsum. As in the case of gypsum, a small expansion results from the outward thrust of growing crystals. The material is also able to undergo hygroscopic expansion if placed in contact with moisture during setting. Moisture adversely affects the unmixed material and the container should always be kept closed when not in use.

The use of a colloidal solution of silica instead of water for mixing with the powder has the dual effect of increasing the setting expansion and strengthening the set material.

On heating the investment prior to casting, mould enlargement occurs by both thermal expansion and inversion of the silica. Thermal expansion is greater for the colloidal silica-mixed materials than for the water-mixed materials. At a temperature of about 300°C ammonia and water are liberated by the reaction:

$$2(Mg \cdot NH_4 \cdot PO_4 \cdot 6H_2O) \rightarrow$$
$$Mg_2 \cdot P_2O_7 + 2NH_3 + 13\ H_2O$$

At higher temperature some of the remaining phosphate reacts with silica forming complex silicophosphates. These cause a significant increase in the strength of the material at the casting temperature.

5.4 Properties of investment materials

Thermal stability One of the primary requirements of an investment is that it should retain its integrity at the casting temperature and have sufficient strength to withstand the stresses set up when the molten alloy enters the investment mould.

Gypsum-bonded investments decompose above 1200°C by interaction of silica with calcium sulphate to liberate sulphur trioxide gas.

$$CaSO_4 + SiO_2 \rightarrow CaSiO_3 + SO_3$$

This not only causes severe weakening of the investment but would lead to the incorporation of porosity into the castings. Thus, gypsum-bonded materials are generally restricted to use with those alloys which are cast well below 1200°C. This includes the majority of the gold alloys and some of the lower melting, base metal alloys. The majority of base metal alloys, however, have higher casting temperatures and require the use of a silica-bonded or phosphate-bonded material.

Another reaction which may take place on heating gypsum-bonded investments is that between calcium sulphate and carbon.

$$CaSO_4 + 4C \rightarrow CaS + 4CO$$

The carbon may be derived from the residue left after burning out of the wax pattern or may be present as graphite in the investment. Further reaction can occur liberating sulphur dioxide.

$$3CaSO_4 + CaS \rightarrow 4CaO + 4SO_2$$

These reactions occur above 700°C and their effects can be minimized by 'heat soaking' the investment mould at the casting temperature to allow the reaction to be completed before casting commences.

The presence of an oxalate in some investments reduces the effects of gypsum decomposition products by liberating carbon dioxide at elevated temperatures.

Phosphate- and silica-bonded materials have sufficient strength at the high temperatures used for casting base metal alloys. The strength of the phosphate-bonded materials is aided by the formation of silicophosphates on heating.

The cohesive strength of the phosphate investments is such that they do not have to be contained in a metal casting ring. The material is generally allowed to set inside a plastic ring which is removed before heating.

Porosity The gypsum-bonded and phosphate bonded materials are sufficiently porous to allow escape of air and other gases from the mould during casting. The silica-bonded materials, on the other hand, are so closely packed that they are virtually porosity-free and there is a danger of 'back pressure' building up which will cause the mould to be incompletely filled or the castings to be porous. These problems can be overcome by making vents in the investment which prevent the pressure from increasing.

Compensating expansion The accuracy of fit of a casting depends primarily on the ability of the investment material to compensate for the shrinkage of the alloy which occurs on casting. The magnitude of the shrinkage varies widely but is of the order of 1·4 percent for most gold alloys, 2·0 percent for Ni/Cr alloys and 2·3 percent for Co/Cr alloys.

The compensating expansion is achieved by a combination of setting expansion, thermal expansion and the expansion which occurs when silica undergoes *inversion* at elevated temperatures.

Hygroscopic expansion can be used to supplement the setting expansion of gypsum-bonded materials. This is also possible for phosphate-bonded materials but is rarely used in practice for these products.

The setting expansion of a typical gypsum-bonded material is of the order of 0·3 percent

Table 5.1 Applications of the various types of investment material

Investment	Primary use
Dental plaster or stone	Mould for acrylic dentures
Gypsum-bonded materials	Mould for gold casting alloys
Silica-bonded materials Phosphate-bonded materials	Moulds for base metal casting alloys

which may be increased to around 1·3 percent by hygroscopic expansion.

The degree of thermal expansion depends on the nature of the silica refractory used in the investment and the temperature to which the mould is heated. Investments containing cristobalite undergo greater thermal expansion than those containing quartz, as shown in Fig. 5.3 for a gypsum-bonded material. If hygroscopic expansion has been used to achieve expansion it is likely that the magnitude of the thermal expansion required will be relatively small. When thermal expansion is used as the primary means of achieving compensation a cristobalite-containing investment mould heated to around 700°C is required.

Silica-bonded investments undergo a slight contraction during setting and the early stages of heating. This is due to the nature of the setting reaction and the subsequent loss of water and alcohol from the material. Continued heating causes considerable expansion due to the close-packed nature of the silica particles. A maximum linear expansion of approximately 1·6 percent is reached at a temperature of about 600°C.

For phosphate-bonded materials a combined setting expansion and thermal expansion of around 2 percent is normal, provided the special silica liquid is used with the investment.

It can be seen that whereas gypsum-bonded investments adequately compensate for the casting shrinkage of gold alloys the same cannot be said for the silica-bonded and phosphate-bonded investments when used with some base metal alloys. It would appear that the large casting shrinkage of the base metal alloys may be a problem which cannot readily be overcome with presently available investments. It should be remembered, however, that further compensation may take place during other stages in the production of the casting. A small contraction of the impression, for example, may give the required compensation.

5.5 Applications

Table 5.1 gives the primary applications of the three main groups of investment materials.

6

Metals and Alloys

6.1 Introduction

Metals and alloys have many uses in dentistry. Steel alloys are commonly used for the construction of instruments and of wires for orthodontics. Gold alloys and alloys containing chromium are used for making crowns, inlays and denture bases whilst dental amalgam, an alloy containing mercury, is the most widely used dental filling material.

With the exception of mercury, metals are generally hard and lustrous at ambient temperatures, and have crystalline structures in which the atoms are closely packed together. Metals are opaque and are good conductors of both heat and electricity.

The shaping of metals and alloys for dental use can be accomplished by one of three methods, namely, casting, cold working or amalgamation. Casting involves heating the material until it becomes molten, when it can be forced into an investment mould which has been prepared from a wax pattern. Cold working involves mechanical shaping of the metal at relatively low temperatures, taking advantage of the high values of ductility and malleability possessed by many metals. Some alloys can be mixed with mercury to form a plastic mass which gradually hardens by a chemical reaction followed by crystallization. The material is shaped by packing it into a tooth cavity whilst still in the plastic state. This specific technique of shaping by amalgamation is dealt with in detail in the chapter devoted to dental amalgam (Chap. 21).

6.2 Structure and properties of metals

Crystal structure

Metals usually have crystalline structures in the solid state. When a molten metal or alloy is cooled, the solidification process is one of crystallization and is initiated at specific sites called nuclei. The nuclei are generally formed from impurities within the molten mass of metal (Fig. 6.1a). Crystals grow as dendrites, which can be described as three-dimensional, branched network structures emanating from the central nucleus (Fig. 6.1b). Crystal growth continues until all the material has solidified and all the dendritic crystals are in contact (Fig. 6.1c). Each crystal is known as a *grain* and the area between two grains in contact is the *grain boundary*.

After crystallization, the grains have approximately the same dimensions in each direction, measured from the central nucleus. They are not perfectly spherical or cubic however, nor do they conform to any other geometric shape. They are said to have an *equiaxed* grain structure. A change from an equiaxed structure to one in which the grains have a more elongated, fibrous structure can cause important changes in mechanical properties.

The atoms within each grain are arranged in a regular three-dimensional lattice. There are several possible arrangements such as cubic, body-centred cubic and face-centred cubic as shown in Fig. 6.2. The arrangement adopted by any one crystal depends on specific factors such as atomic radius and charge distributions on the atoms. Although there is a tendency towards a perfect crystal structure, occasional defects occur, as illustrated, two-dimensionally, in Fig. 6.3. Such defects are normally referred to as *dislocations* and their occurrence has an effect on the *ductility* of the metal or alloy. When the material is placed under a sufficiently high stress the dislocation is able to move through the lattice until it reaches a grain boundary. The plane along which the dislocation moves is called a *slip plane* and the stress required to initiate movement is the elastic limit.

In practical terms, the application of a stress greater than the elastic limit causes the material to be permanently deformed as a result of movement of dislocations. Depending upon the circumstances, this can be a disadvantage or, alternatively, may be used to advantage, as in the formation of wires.

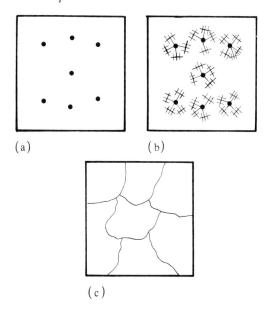

(a)   (b)

(c)

Fig. 6.1 Diagram illustrating crystallization of a metal (a) from nuclei, (b) through dendritic growth, (c) to form grains.

Grain boundaries form a natural barrier to the movement of dislocations. The concentration of grain boundaries increases as the grain size decreases. Metals with finer grain structure are generally harder and have higher values of elastic limit than those with coarser grain structure. Hence it can be seen that material properties can be controlled to some extent by controlling the grain size.

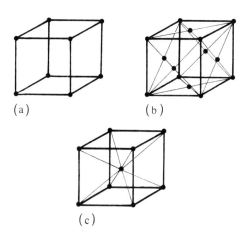

(a)   (b)

(c)

Fig. 6.2 Some possible arrangements of atoms in metals and alloys: (a) cubic structure; (b) face-centred cubic; (c) body-centred cubic.

A fine grain structure can be achieved by rapid cooling of the molten metal or alloy following casting. This process, often referred to as *quenching*, ensures that many nuclei of crystallization are formed, resulting in a large number of relatively small grains as shown in Fig. 6.4a. Slow cooling causes relatively few nuclei to be formed which results in a larger grain size as shown in Fig. 6.4b. Some metals and alloys are said to have a *refined grain structure*. This is normally a fine grain structure which is achieved by *seeding* the molten ma-

(a)

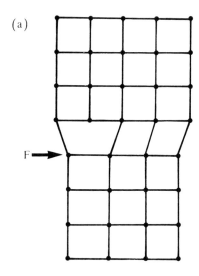

F

(b)

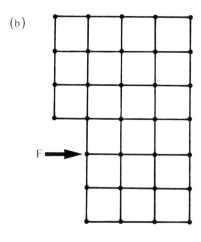

F

Fig. 6.3 (a) Simplified, diagrammatic indication of an imperfection in a crystal structure. (b) Under the influence of sufficient force atoms may move to establish a more perfect arrangement.

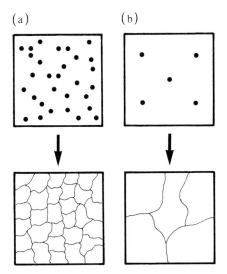

Fig. 6.4 Control of metallic grain size by controlling the rate of cooling from the melt. (a) Rapid cooling — more nuclei, smaller grains. (b) Slow cooling — fewer nuclei, larger grains.

terial with an additive metal which forms nuclei for crystallization.

Cold working

In the previous section it was mentioned that permanent deformation takes place on the application of a sufficiently high force, due to the movement of dislocations along slip planes. For an applied tensile force the maximum degree of extension is a measure of the *ductility* of the metal or alloy. For an applied compressive force the maximum degree of compression is a measure of *malleability*. These changes occur when the stress is greater than the elastic limit and at relatively low temperatures. Such *cold working* not only produces a change in microstructure, with dislocations becoming concentrated at grain boundaries, but also a change in grain shape. The grains are no longer equiaxed but take up a more *fibrous* structure (Fig. 6.5a). The properties of the material are altered, becoming harder and stronger with a higher value of elastic limit. The ductility or malleability is decreased because the potential for further cold working is reduced. Cold working is sometimes referred to as *work hardening* due to the effect on mechanical properties. When mechanical work is carried out on a metal or alloy at a more elevated temperature it is possible for the metal object to change shape

without any alteration in grain shape or mechanical properties (Fig. 6.5b). The temperature below which work hardening is possible is termed the *recrystallization temperature*. Some examples of cold working in dentistry include:

(1) The formation of wires, in which an alloy is forced through a series of circular dies of gradually decreasing diameter. The resulting fibrous grain structure is responsible for the special 'springy' properties possessed by most wires,

(2) The bending of wires or clasps during the construction and alteration of appliances,

(3) The swaging of stainless steel denture bases.

Since metals and alloys have finite values of ductility or malleability there is a limit to the amount of cold working which can be carried out. Attempts to carry out further cold working beyond this limit may result in fracture. This limitation should be remembered when carrying out alterations to clasps constructed from low-ductility alloys.

If a cold-worked metal or alloy with a fibrous grain structure is heated to above its recrystallization temperature it gradually reverts to an equiaxed form and becomes softer with a lower value of elastic limit but a higher ductility. Hence, recrystallization can be used as a softening heat treatment. In many applications of wrought alloys however, it is something which must be avoided because of the adverse effect on mechanical properties. If the material is maintained above the recrystallization temperature for sufficient time, diffusion of atoms across grain boundaries may occur, leading to *grain growth*. The effect of grain size on mechanical pro-

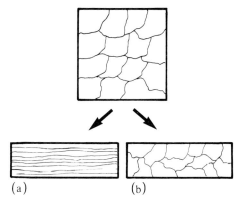

Fig. 6.5 Mechanical work carried out on a sample of metal or alloy. (a) Below the recrystallization temperature — produces a fibrous grain structure. (b) Above the recrystallization temperature — retains an equiaxed grain structure.

perties has already been discussed and it is clear that grain growth should be avoided if the properties are not to be adversely affected.

Cold working may cause the formation of internal stresses within a metal object. If these stresses are gradually relieved they may cause distortion which could lead to loss of fit of, for example, an orthodontic appliance. For certain metals and alloys the internal stresses can be wholly or partly eliminated by using a low temperature heat treatment referred to as *stress relief annealing*. This heat treatment is carried out well below the recrystallization temperature and has no deleterious effect on mechanical properties since the fibrous grain structure is maintained.

6.3 Structure and properties of alloys

An alloy is a mixture of two or more metals. Mixtures of two metals are termed binary alloys, mixtures of three metals ternary alloys etc. The term *alloy system* refers to all possible compositions of an alloy. For example the silver−copper system refers to all alloys with compositions ranging between 100 percent silver and 100 percent copper.

In the molten state metals usually show mutual solubility, one within another. When the molten mixture is cooled to below the melting point one of four things can occur:

(1) The component metals may remain soluble in each other forming a *solid solution*. The solid solution may take one of three forms. It may be a *random solid solution* in which the component metal atoms occupy random sites in a common crystal lattice. Another possibility is the formation of an *ordered solid solution* in which component metal atoms occupy specific sites within a common crystal lattice. The third type of solid solution is the *interstitial solid solution* in which, for binary alloys, the primary lattice sites are occupied by one metal atom and the atoms of the second component do not occupy lattice sites but lie within the interstices of the lattice. This is normally found where the atomic radius of one component is much smaller than that of the other.

Solid solutions are generally harder, stronger and have higher values of elastic limit than the pure metals from which they are derived. This explains why pure metals are rarely used. The hardening effect, known as *solution hardening*, is thought to be due to the fact that atoms of different atomic radii within the same lattice form a mechanical

resistance to the movement of dislocations along slip planes.

(2) The component metals may be completely insoluble in the solid state. Examination of a binary alloy of two metals, A and B, showing this behaviour reveals the presence of some areas containing pure metal A and others containing pure metal B. This type of alloy is susceptible to electrolytic corrosion, as described on p.25, particularly if the component metals have widely differing electrochemical potentials.

(3) The two metals may be partially soluble in the solid state. For metals A and B two distinct phases exist within the solid state. One phase consists of a solid solution of metal B in metal A, whilst the other phase consists of a solid solution of A in B.

(4) If the two metals show a particular affinity for one another they may form intermetallic compounds with precise chemical formulation (e.g. Ag_3Sn). Since intermetallic compounds have specific valence requirements there are fewer crystal imperfections and the potential for movement along slip planes is reduced. Such materials therefore tend to be relatively hard and brittle with low ductility.

Most alloys have properties which are specific to the particular system being considered. The general principles discussed for metals in the previous section, however, also hold true for most alloy systems. Hence, the grain size of alloys can be controlled by the rate of cooling from the melt. Alloys can be work hardened and they undergo recrystallization and grain growth under the correct conditions.

6.4 Cooling curves

Metals and alloys are sometimes characterized using cooling curves. The material is heated till molten then allowed to cool and a plot of temperature against time is recorded, as shown in Fig. 6.6. For a pure metal (Fig. 6.6a) the cooling curve displays a distinct plateau region at the melting point (T_m) indicating that temperature remains constant over a period of time during crystallization. With few exceptions, the cooling curves for alloys show no such plateau region (Fig. 6.6b). Crystallization begins at temperature T_1, and is complete at temperature T_2. Hence crystallization takes place over a range of temperatures.

(a)

(b)

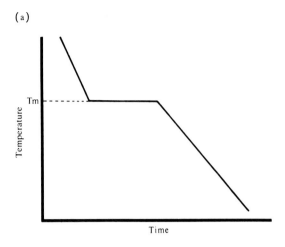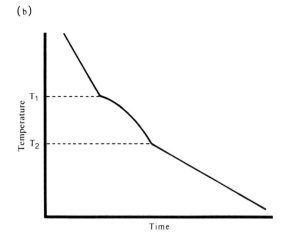

Fig. 6.6 Cooling curves for (a) a pure metal, showing solidification at a fixed temperature and (b) an alloy showing solidification over a range of temperatures.

For a binary solid solution alloy of two metals, A and B, in which the melting point of metal A is greater than that of metal B, the first material to crystallize, at just below temperature T_1, will be rich in the higher melting point metal A, whilst the last material to crystallize, at a temperature just above T_2, is rich in the lower melting point metal B. The result is therefore a concentration gradient within the solidified alloy. The material is said to have a *cored* structure. Such *coring* may influence corrosion resistance since electrolytic cells may be set up on the surface of the alloy between areas of different alloy composition.

If a series of cooling curves for alloys of different composition within a given alloy system are available a *phase diagram* can be constructed from which many important predictions regarding coring and other structural variations can be made.

6.5 **Phase diagrams**

The temperature range over which an alloy crystallizes can readily be obtained from the cooling curve, as illustrated in Fig. 6.6b. If the temperatures T_1 and T_2 are obtained over a range of compositions for an alloy system and their values plotted against percentage composition, a useful graph emerges. This is illustrated in Fig. 6.7 for a hypothetical solid solution alloy of metals A and B. The melting points of the pure metals are indicated by the temperatures TmA and TmB. The upper and lower

temperature limits of the crystallization range, T_1 and T_2, are shown for four alloys ranging in composition from 80 percent A/20 percent B to 20 percent A/80 percent B.

The phase diagram is completed by joining together all the T_1 points and all the T_2 points, together with the melting points of the pure metals, TmA and TmB. At temperatures in the region above the top line, known as the *liquidus line*, the alloy is totally liquid. At temperatures in the region below the bottom line, known as the *solidus line*, the alloy is totally solid. At temperatures in the region between the solidus and liquidus lines the alloy consists of a mixture of solid and liquid. The composition of the solid and liquid phases at any temperature between T_1 and T_2 can be predicted with the aid of the phase diagram.

Solid solution phase diagrams

Fig. 6.7 shows how the phase diagram for a binary solid solution alloy is constructed. The diagram is redrawn in Fig. 6.8 in order to illustrate how it may be used to predict some of the characteristics of the alloy. Consider, for example, an alloy of composition X (approximately 60 percent A and 40 percent B). This alloy may be rendered completely molten by heating it to a temperature above T_L which represents the liquidus temperature for that particular composition. If the alloy is cooled from above T_L it remains molten until the temperature T_L is

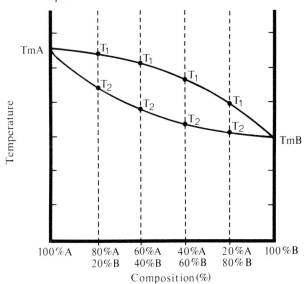

Fig. 6.7 Phase diagram of a solid solution alloy constructed from a series of cooling curves (Fig. 6.6). The temperatures T_1 and T_2 are obtained from experiments using alloys of varying composition.

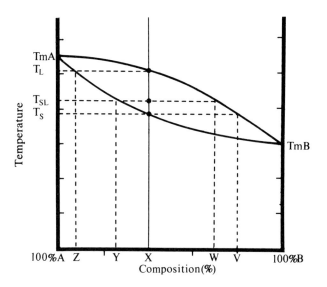

Fig. 6.8 Diagram illustrating how a solid solution phase diagram can be used to predict or explain certain alloy characteristics.

reached, when the first solid begins to form. The composition of the first solid to form is given by drawing a horizontal line or *tie line* to intersect the solidus. In this case, drawing such a tie line reveals that the first solid to form has composition Z (approximately 90 percent A/10 percent B). As the alloy is cooled further, more crystallization occurs and between temperatures T_L and T_S a mixture of solid and liquid exists. Selecting one temperature, T_{SL}, within this region, the composition of both solid and liquid can be predicted, by noting where the tie line intersects both solidus and liquidus. Thus, at temperature T_{SL} the composition of the

solid is Y (approximately 80 percent A/20 percent B) and the composition of the remaining liquid is W (approximately 75 percent B/25 percent A). On further cooling, the alloy becomes completely solid at temperature T_S. The last liquid to crystallize has the composition V (approximately 80 percent B/20 percent A). This confirms the previous observation that for solid solution alloys a cored structure exists in which the first material to crystallize is rich in the metal with the higher melting point (A), whilst the last material to solidify is rich in the other metal (B). In the case of the alloy described, the variation in composition within the solidified alloy ranges

(a)

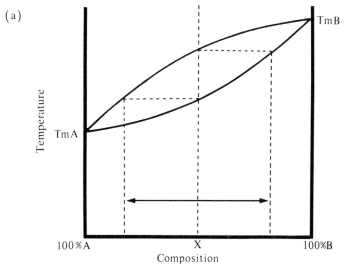

Fig. 6.9 Diagram to show how the extent of coring depends on the separation of solidus and liquidus lines. (a) Solidus and liquidus widely separated. Extensive coring as illustrated by arrows. (b) Solidus and liquidus closer together resulting in less extensive coring.

(b)

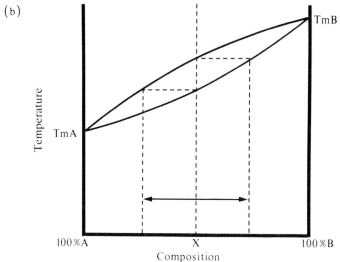

from 90 percent A/10 percent B at one extreme to 80 percent B/20 percent A at the other. An indication of the degree of coring is given by the separation of the solidus and liquidus lines on the phase diagram. The potential for coring is greater when there is wide separation of solidus and liquidus lines as shown in Fig. 6.9.

The previous discussion describes what happens when a solid solution alloy is cooled rapidly, as occurs for example, during casting. With slow cooling the crystallization process is accompanied by diffusion and a random distribution of atoms results, with no coring. Rapid cooling quickly denies the alloy the energy and mobility required for diffusion of atoms to occur and the cored struc-

ture is 'locked in' at low temperatures. Reducing the cooling rate as a means of eliminating coring would be self-defeating since it would produce an alloy with large grain size which, of course, would have inferior mechanical properties.

Since coring may markedly reduce the corrosion resistance of some alloys, a heat treatment is sometimes used to eliminate the cored structure. Such a heat treatment is termed a *homogenization* heat treatment. This involves heating the alloy to a temperature just below the solidus temperature for a few minutes to allow diffusion of atoms and the establishment of a homogeneous structure. The alloy is then normally quenched in order to prevent grain growth from occurring.

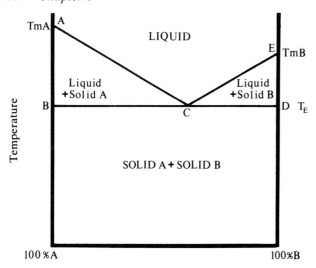

Fig. 6.10 Phase diagram of an alloy of two metals (A and B) which are completely insoluble in the solid phase. The alloy with composition equivalent to point C is termed a eutectic alloy. This type of phase diagram is sometimes called a eutectic phase diagram.

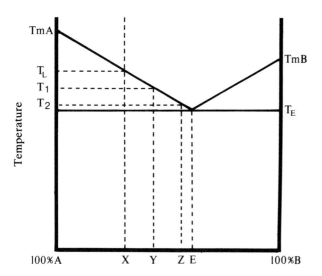

Fig. 6.11 Diagram illustrating how a eutectic phase diagram can be utilized.

Eutectic phase diagrams

It has already been pointed out that some metals are completely insoluble in the solid phase and an alloy of such metals consists of a mixture of grains of the pure metal components. Phase diagrams may be constructed by exactly the same technique as that described for solid solutions — by constructing cooling curves and noting the temperatures at which crystallization commences and is complete. Such a phase diagram for a hypothetical alloy of two metals, A and B, is shown in Fig. 6.10. The liquidus line is given by joining points A, C and E, whilst the solidus is given by A B C D E. The temperatures TmA and TmB are again the melting points of the pure metals A and B. In the two triangular regions between the solidus and liquidus lines a mixture of solid and liquid exists. The solid is always one of the pure metals. To the right of point C it is always pure B and to the left of point C is always pure A. The alloy with composition corresponding to point C is called the *eutectic alloy* and is of particular interest since it crystallizes at a given temperature and not over a range of temperatures. In this respect, the eutectic alloy behaves in a similar fashion to a pure metal. Alloys with composition close to the eutectic composition have narrow melting ranges and melting points considerably lower than those of the component pure metals. For these reasons they are often used as solders.

The eutectic phase diagram can be used to predict composition changes during crystallization in just the same way as the solid solution diagram was used. For the most simple case of the eutectic alloy, it solidifies at temperature T_E to give a mixture of metals A and B. Fig. 6.11 illustrates what happens during crystallization for an alloy, X, not having the eutectic composition. On cooling, crystallization begins at temperature T_1. The intersection of the horizontal tie line with the solidus indicates that the first material to crystallize is pure metal A. At temperature T_1 the alloy lies in the region between solidus and liquidus lines, indicating that a mixture of solid and liquid exists. The compositions of solid and liquid are given by the points of intersection of the tie line with the solidus and liquidus lines. Thus it can be seen that at T_1 the solid formed is still pure metal A whilst the remaining liquid has composition Y. On cooling further to temperature T_2, the solid is still pure metal A but the remaining liquid has composition Z, very close to the eutectic composition (E). Finally, on reaching temperature T_E the eutectic mixture of metals remaining in the liquid phase crystallize out.

Hence, a simplified explanation of what happens during cooling is that one of the pure metals crystallizes until the remaining mixture of molten metals has a composition equivalent to the eutectic. At this stage the remaining metals crystallize together.

The solidified alloy consists of a mixture of insoluble metals which often has inferior corrosion resistance due to the potential for the establishment of electrolytic cells on the surface of the alloy.

Other alloy systems

The preceding discussion of alloy cooling curves and the formation of phase diagrams for solid solutions and eutectics illustrates how important information on alloy systems can be gathered and utilized. Every alloy system has its own distinctive phase diagram which can be used to characterize that system. The principles behind the use of such diagrams are the same as those described here.

In the following chapters, specific alloy systems used in dentistry are discussed and some of their properties are illustrated with the aid of phase diagrams where necessary. In some cases, structural transitions of alloys occur, not during crystallization, but within the solid phase. Such solid–solid transitions complicate phase diagrams by adding more lines but do not alter the way in which the diagrams are used.

7 Gold and Gold Alloys

7.1 Introduction

In the 'as cast' condition, pure gold is too soft to maintain its shape under the forces of mastication. Its strength and hardness can be greatly improved by either cold working or alloying.

Gold is very malleable and ductile and can be readily cold worked. This characteristic is utilized in the restoration of teeth using pure gold fillings. Alloys of gold are commonly used for cast restorations. The use of wrought gold wires is dealt with in a separate chapter dealing with wrought alloys.

7.2 Pure gold fillings (cohesive gold)

When two pieces of pure gold are pressed together, metallic bonds are formed at their point of contact and the gold is welded together, without the application of heat. This property of *cold welding* is utilized when building up a pure gold filling. The surfaces of the two pieces of gold must be perfectly clean to allow intimate contact and the applied force must be great enough to encourage the formation of bonds.

Cohesive gold is normally used in the form of a very thin gold sheet or 'foil', approximately 0·001 mm thick. On condensation into the prepared cavity, each layer of foil becomes welded to the material already condensed. It is normal practice to heat the gold foil to about 250°C in an electric furnace or a gas flame before use to remove any adsorbed grease or gases which would prevent efficient welding. The tooth to be filled must be isolated from the saliva and thoroughly dried to avoid contamination during condensation.

Condensation or 'plugging' of the gold may be carried out by hand, with an automatic mallet, or by the application of a mechanical vibrator. The use of an automatic mallet involves the application of a relatively large force at infrequent intervals, whereas a pneumatic or electrically driven condenser delivers much lighter, but more frequent blows. Care must be taken not to overheat the filling and cause damage to the pulp. The tooth and its supporting structures must withstand the fairly harsh treatment they receive during condensation without becoming damaged. Fortunately, both the dentine and periodontal membrane are fairly resilient.

The mechanical properties of the pure gold filling depend on the amount of cold working carried out on the material. The degree of work hardening depends on the pressure applied during condensation and the length of time for which the material is condensed. Practical limitations of time and the pressure which can be tolerated by the patient restrict the hardness of the pure gold filling to values similar to those for the softer (type I) casting gold alloys.

The advantages of the gold foil filling are that it is perfectly corrosion resistant and does not rely on a relatively soluble cement lute for retention. In cavities where the filling is surrounded by tooth substance, or where there is little or no opposing force, the mechanical properties are adequate and the pure gold filling offers a very durable restoration.

7.3 Casting gold alloys

An indication of the composition of the casting gold alloys is given in Table 7.1. It can be seen that the gold content or *nobility* decreases on going from the type I (soft) alloy to the type IV (extra hard) alloy. Nobility of gold alloys is often indicated by either a *carat* value or a *fineness* value. The carat value indicates the number of parts by weight of gold in 24 parts of alloy. Thus, a type II alloy containing 75 percent gold has a carat value of 18. The fineness value indicates the number of parts by weight of gold in 1000 parts of alloy. The type II alloy would have a fineness value of 750.

Table 7.1 Typical compositions of casting gold alloys

Type	Au percentage	Ag percentage	Cu percentage	Pt/Pd percentage	Zn percentage
I (soft)	85	11	3	—	1
II (medium)	75	12	10	2	1
III (hard)	70	14	10	5	1
IV (extra hard)	65	13	15	6	1

The increase in hardness observed when nobility decreases is primarily due to the *solution hardening* effect of the alloying metals which all form solid solutions with gold. The types III and IV alloys can be further hardened by heat treatments.

The presence of significant quantities of platinum and palladium, as in the types III and IV alloys, not only causes considerable solution hardening but also leads to a widening of the separation between the solidus and liquidus lines of the solid solution phase diagram. The result of this is an increase in *coring* as explained on p.49. The cored structure can be removed by carrying out a *homogenization* heat treatment. Platinum and palladium also significantly increase the melting point and recrystallization temperature of gold alloys, a fact which can be used to advantage when selecting alloys for components which may require soldering.

Zinc, which is present to a concentration of about 1 percent in most alloys, acts as a *scavenger* during casting. It is the most chemically reactive of all the metals used and becomes preferentially oxidized at the high temperatures of casting. The resulting zinc oxide slag can be removed from the molten alloy.

Table 7.2 gives an indication of the comparative properties of the four types of casting gold alloys. Moving through the series from type I to type IV, there is an increase in hardness, strength and proportional limit. The corrosion resistance decreases as the gold content is reduced, although for prac-

tical purposes all of the alloys may be considered adequate from this point of view. Ductility and malleability also decrease when the gold content is reduced.

The variation in alloy properties with composition is reflected in the applications for which the materials are chosen. The relatively soft, type I alloys are used for inlays which are well supported by tooth substance and which do not have to resist large masticatory forces. The high values of ductility of these alloys enables them to be burnished — a process which improves the marginal fit of the inlay and increases surface hardness. The need to improve the fit of inlays by burnishing has decreased with improvements in casting accuracy.

The type II alloys are the most widely used alloys for inlays. They have superior mechanical properties when compared with the type I materials, though at the expense of a slight decrease in ductility.

The type III (hard) alloys are used where there is less support from tooth substance and when opposing stresses are likely to be relatively high. Examples of the use of these materials include the production of crowns, bridges and inlays for high stress areas such as class II cavities in molars. The high platinum and/or palladium content of the type III alloys, leading to a higher melting point, is beneficial when constructing components for bridges which are joined by soldering.

Type IV alloys are used exclusively for construc-

Table 7.2 Comparative properties of casting gold alloys

Type	Hardness	Proportional limit	Strength	Ductility	Corrosion resistance
I II III IV	↑ Increases ↓	↑ Increases ↓	↑ Increases ↓	↑ Decreases ↓	↑ Decreases ↓

ting components of partial dentures and for this reason are normally referred to as *partial denture casting alloys*. Partial dentures normally have clasps or other devices for retaining the denture. These must be flexible enough to engage undercuts in standing teeth but have sufficiently high values of proportional limit such that they do not become distorted. The type IV gold alloys possess this useful combination of properties. In addition, the alloys have sufficient ductility in the softened state to allow slight adjustments to be made. Attempts to carry out adjustments on a heat hardened alloy may lead to fracture due to the decrease in ductility which accompanies hardening.

The connectors of partial dentures, be they bars or plates, should be rigid and resist distortion. Whereas the proportional limit of type IV gold alloys is sufficiently high to resist distortion, the connectors must be constructed in fairly thick section in order to produce sufficient rigidity due to the relatively low value of modulus of elasticity of these alloys. Some base metal denture casting alloys have higher values of modulus and from this point of view are more satisfactory for producing connectors.

7.4 Hardening heat treatments (theoretical considerations)

The type III (hard) and type IV (extra hard) casting gold alloys can be further hardened by heat treatments. The hardening process can be explained by consideration of the phase diagrams for the silver−copper and gold−copper systems. Hardening heat treatments are not beneficial for the types I and II alloys because they contain insufficient quantities of copper and silver.

Silver−copper system

The silver−copper system is a good example of an alloy in which the component metals are only partially soluble in the solid state. The solidified alloy consists of a mixture of two solid solutions, one in which small quantities of copper are dissolved in silver (called the α solid solution) and one in which small quantities of silver are dissolved in copper (the β solid solution).

The phase diagram for the silver−copper system is shown in Fig. 7.1. In some respects it resembles the eutectic phase diagram given in Fig. 6.10. The solidus is defined by the line A B E C D, whilst the liquidus is given by A E D. The compositional limits of the α and β solid solutions are denoted by the areas marked α and β on the phase diagram. The lines B F and C G are termed *solvus lines* and indicate the decreasing solubility of copper in silver and silver in copper as the temperature decreases. Thus the solubility of copper in silver is around 9 percent at 780°C (the eutectic temperature) but only around 2 percent at 400°C. This relationship between solubility and temperature is normal for any system of limited solubility.

When an alloy of the eutectic composition (72 percent Ag/28 percent Cu) is cooled from the molten state it undergoes solidification at a constant temperature, equivalent to point E on the phase diagram. The solid formed is a mixture of α and β solid solutions in which the α has composition equivalent to point B (approximately 9 percent Cu/91 percent Ag) and the β has composition equivalent to point C (approximately 8 percent Ag/92 percent Cu). An alloy with slightly more copper than the eutectic composition solidifies to give the eutectic mixture plus additional β solid solution. An alloy with slightly more silver than the eutectic composition solidifies to give the eutectic mixture and additional α solid solution. Using the lines it can be shown that during crystallization the excess

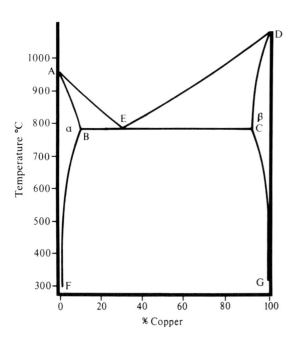

Fig. 7.1 Phase diagram of the silver−copper system.

solid solution crystallizes first and that the eutectic mixture is always the last to crystallize.

If the alloy has either less than 9 percent or greater than 92 percent copper then the solid formed is either α *or* β solid solution — no eutectic mixture is formed.

When casting, generally, alloys are cooled rapidly to encourage the formation of a fine grain structure. At low temperatures the alloys become rigid and atomic diffusions become difficult if not impossible. The structure of the alloy which was formed during crystallization becomes 'frozen' into the alloy at room temperature. Despite the fact that the solubilities of silver in copper and copper in silver are negligible at room temperature, there exist, within the eutectic mixture, α and β solid solutions in which 9 percent copper remains dissolved in silver and 8 percent silver remains dissolved in copper. If diffusion were possible, there would be a tendency for copper to precipitate from the α solid solution and silver to precipitate from the β solid solution.

It is possible to heat the alloy to a temperature at which the solubility is exceeded but at which atomic diffusions are possible. In the temperature range 300–600°C slow diffusion of copper atoms can occur. Given sufficient time in this temperature range copper would begin to precipitate from the α solid solution. Well before any precipitated phase can be observed however, a significant hardening of the alloy takes place, presumably because the diffusing atoms have effectively prevented movement of slip planes. This forms the basis of the *precipitation hardening* procedure used for type III and type IV casting gold alloys.

Gold—copper system

Gold and copper form a continuous series of solid solutions over the whole range of compositions. The solid solutions are random-substitutional solid solutions with face-centred cubic lattices (Fig. 7.2).

The phase diagram for the gold—copper system is shown in Fig. 7.3. It can be seen that the solidus and liquidus are close together and almost coincide at point M. Two other areas on the phase diagram, at compositions between 40 percent gold and 90 percent gold, indicate regions in which the alloys are capable of undergoing a solid—solid transition to form an ordered rather than disordered lattice. The ordered lattice, in which gold and copper take up specific lattice sites, is often referred to as a superlattice.

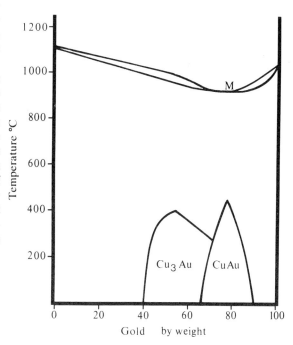

Fig. 7.3 Simplified phase diagram of the gold—copper system.

Formation of the superlattice requires that an atomic rearrangement must take place by diffusion of atoms. This cannot occur at normal temperatures since there is insufficient energy in the system to allow diffusion to occur. Consider, for example, an alloy containing 75 percent gold which lies within one of the areas of interest. If this alloy is heated to a temperature in the region 200–400°C, sufficient energy is imparted to the system to allow

Disordered

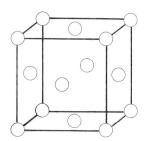

Fig. 7.2 Disordered, face-centred cubic, gold—copper alloy. Circles represent either gold or copper.

atomic diffusions to occur, atoms take up their preferred sites and the superlattice is formed. In this case the superlattice has the formula CuAu and the superlattice has an ordered tetragonal structure as shown in Fig. 7.4. In alloys containing 40−60 percent gold an ordered superlattice, based on the formula Cu_3Au, is formed. The change in size and shape of the gold−copper lattice sets up a resistance to the movement of slip planes within the multi-component casting gold alloy which results in a significant increase in hardness and strength and a reduction in ductility. Heat treatments which are used to carry out this hardening procedure are termed *order hardening* heat treatments.

Ordered

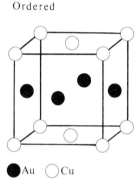

●Au ○Cu

Fig. 7.4 Ordered, tetragonal structure of a heat-treated, gold−copper alloy containing 75 percent gold.

7.5 **Heat treatments (practical considerations)**
On melting the alloy prior to casting, any metallographic structure which it possessed as an ingot is lost and a new crystal structure is created as the metal 'freezes' inside the mould.

It is important to quench the gold alloy castings before they cool to the range of temperatures within which heat hardening takes place. An alloy which is allowed to cool slowly to room temperature will undergo both precipitation and order hardening prematurely. Before any alteration in shape of such a casting is attempted, it must be softened by cooling rapidly from above 600°C. Normal casting procedure is to leave the mould until the gold, visible in the sprues of the casting, is no longer at red heat. This indicates that the internal metal temperature is about 600°C. The mould is then plunged into cold water in order to chill the metal quickly and cause disintegration of the mould. Rapid cooling also helps to ensure a fine grain structure.

The casting is then cleaned and when platinum or palladium are present a homogenization heat treatment is carried out to remove coring. This involves heating to 700°C for ten minutes, then quenching. The casting is then polished and its fit in the mouth is checked. Any minor adjustments, such as bending of clasps etc., are made at this stage whilst the alloy is still in the softened state. If adjustments are made, a low temperature *stress relief anneal* should be carried out.

The hardening heat treatment may then be carried out with type III and type IV alloys by heating the casting to above 450°C and allowing it to cool slowly until its temperature has dropped to about 200°C, then quenching. This takes about 20 minutes for an average-sized casting. The precise details of the heat treatment vary from one alloy to another and the manufacturer's instructions should be followed. The procedures are designed such that hardening by both precipitation and ordering can occur.

Following hardening the casting is repolished and, in the case of a denture, the teeth are added in order to complete the job.

Ideally, all hardening and softening heat treatments should be carried out in a pyrometrically controlled furnace. The castings should be supported by sand or another refractory material in order to prevent 'sag' at elevated temperatures.

7.6 **Low gold-content alloys**
Large increases in the price of gold have led to the development and increased use of alloys with lower gold content than those described previously. Some alloys contain as little as 10 percent gold but more normally a gold content of around 45−50 percent is used. They have a high palladium content which imparts a characteristic 'whitish' colour to the alloys.

The properties of the low-gold alloys vary from one product to another but are broadly similar to those of the type III and type IV casting gold alloys, with one main exception. The ductility of these alloys tends to be significantly lower than for conventional gold alloys. A typical type III gold alloy can undergo an extension of 20 percent before fracture, whereas a typical low-gold alloy can extend only 2 percent. This must be remembered when making alterations to clasps of partial dentures constructed from low-gold alloys. Any attempt to carry out extensive bending is likely to result in fracture.

The casting techniques and equipment used for low-gold alloys are similar to those used for conventional gold alloys. This, coupled with their acceptable properties, good clinical performance and lower cost compared to conventional gold alloys, has led to their widespread use.

7.7 Silver–palladium alloys

The silver–palladium alloys contain little or no gold and as their name suggests contain primarily silver and palladium. There is generally a minimum of 25 percent palladium along with small quantities of copper, zinc and indium, in addition to gold which is sometimes present in small quantities.

The silver–palladium alloys have significantly lower density than gold alloys, a factor which may affect castability. For a given volume of casting, there is a lower force generated by the molten alloy during casting. Attention must be paid to details such as casting temperature and mould temperature if the mould is to be adequately filled by the alloy.

Alloys containing large quantities of palladium have a propensity for dissolving oxygen in the molten state which may lead to a porous casting. Care must be taken to avoid overheating or oxidation of the melt during casting.

The properties of the silver–palladium alloys are similar to those of the types III and IV gold alloys with the exception of their lower ductility. The corrosion resistance is not as good as for gold alloys but, provided the palladium content is above 25 percent, the amount of corrosion expected during service is negligible.

These alloys offer a suitable alternative to gold alloys provided that care is taken during casting. They offer a considerable saving in cost when compared to gold alloys.

8 Base Metal Casting Alloys

8.1 Introduction

Base metal alloys contain no gold, silver, platinum or palladium. The two most commonly used base metal alloys in dentistry are the nickel–chromium (Ni/Cr) alloys which are commonly used for crown and bridge casting and the cobalt–chromium (Co/Cr) alloys which are commonly used for partial denture framework castings.

8.2 Composition

Cobalt–chromium alloys (stellites)

These alloys generally contain 35–65 percent cobalt, 20–35 percent chromium, 0–30 percent nickel and trace quantities of other elements such as molybdenum, silicon, beryllium, boron and carbon. Cobalt and nickel are hard, strong metals. The main purpose of the chromium is to further harden the alloy by solution hardening and also to impart corrosion resistance by the *passivating effect*. Chromium exposed at the surface of the alloy rapidly becomes oxidized to form a thin, passive, surface layer of chromic oxide which prevents further attack on the bulk of the alloy. The concentrations of the minor constituents have a greater effect on the physical properties of the alloys than do the relative cobalt–chromium–nickel concentrations. The minor elements are generally added to improve casting and handling characteristics and modify mechanical properties. For example, silicon imparts good casting properties to a nickel-containing alloy and increases its ductility. Likewise, beryllium is added to refine the grain structure and improve the behaviour of base metal alloys during casting. Carbon affects the hardness, strength and ductility of the alloys and the exact concentration of carbon is one of the major factors controlling alloy properties. The carbon forms carbides with other components and its concentration

depends on both the amount added by the manufacturer and that which may be inadvertently introduced during casting if the alloy is melted with an oxyacetylene torch. The presence of too much carbon results in a brittle alloy with very low ductility and an increased danger of fracture.

Nickel–chromium alloys

These alloys vary in composition from one manufacturer to another but generally fall within the range 70–80 percent nickel, 10–25 percent chromium, with small quantities of other elements as described for the Co/Cr alloys.

8.3 Manipulation of base metal casting alloys

The fusion temperatures of the Ni/Cr and Co/Cr alloys vary with composition but are generally in the range 1200–1500°C. This is considerably higher than for the casting gold alloys which rarely have fusion temperatures above 950°C. Melting of gold alloys can readily be achieved using a gas/air mixture. For base metal alloys, however, either an acetylene/oxygen flame or an electrical induction furnace is required. The latter method is to be favoured since it is carried out under more controlled conditions. When using oxyacetylene flames the ratio of oxygen to acetylene must be carefully controlled. Too much oxygen may cause oxidation of the alloy whilst an excess of acetylene produces an increase in the metal carbide content leading to embrittlement.

Investment moulds for Ni/Cr alloys must be capable of maintaining their integrity at the high casting temperatures used. Silica-bonded and phosphate-bonded materials are favoured with the latter product being most widely used. Gypsum-bonded investments decompose above 1200°C to form sulphur dioxide which may be absorbed by the casting, causing embrittlement. This effect can be reduced by the incorporation of oxalate in the investment, however the problem is generally avoided by choosing an investment which is more stable at elevated temperatures.

The density values of base metal alloys are approximately half those of the casting gold alloys. For this reason the thrust developed during casting may be somewhat lower, with the possibility that the casting may not adequately fill the mould. Casting machines used for base metal alloys must therefore be capable of producing extra thrust which overcomes this deficiency. The problem may be aggravated if the investment is not sufficiently porous to allow escape of trapped air and other gases. Careful use of vents and sprues of adequate size is normally sufficient to overcome such problems.

Base metal alloys, and particularly the Co/Cr type, are very hard and consequently difficult to polish. After casting, it is usual to sandblast the metal to remove any surface roughness or adherent investment material. *Electrolytic polishing* may then be carried out. This procedure is essentially the opposite to electroplating. If a rough metal surface is connected as the anode in a bath of strongly acid electrolyte, a current passing between it and the cathode will cause the anode to ionize and lose a surface film of metal. With a suitable electrolyte and the correct current density, the first products of electrolysis will collect in the hollows of the rough metal surface and so prevent further attack in these areas. The prominences of the metal surface will continue to be dissolved and in this way

the contours of the surface are smoothed. Final polishing can be carried out using a high-speed polishing buff.

8.4 Properties

The Co/Cr and Ni/Cr alloys are very hard materials and although this makes the polishing of castings a difficult process the final polished surface is very durable and resistant to scratching.

In addition, fine margins seem less likely to be lost during finishing of a base metal alloy.

Co/Cr alloys have relatively low ductility, a fact which should be remembered when carrying out alterations to partial denture clasps. The ductility may be further reduced if the concentration of carbides becomes increased during melting with an oxyacetylene torch.

Nickel−chromium alloys, on the other hand, are ductile with elongation at fracture values as high as 30 percent. This would suggest that restorations produced from these alloys can be burnished. However, their relatively high proportional limit values indicate that high stresses would be required for effective burnishing.

The proportional limit values of the Co/Cr alloys are somewhat higher than even the Ni/Cr alloys. They are able to withstand high stresses without undergoing permanent deformation.

The Ni/Cr alloys and Co/Cr alloys are both very rigid materials with high modulus of elasticity values.

Table 8.1 Comparative properties of Co/Cr alloys and type IV casting gold alloys for partial dentures

Property (units)	Co/Cr	Type IV gold alloy	Comments
Density (g/cm^3)	8	15	More difficult to produce defect-free castings for Co/Cr alloys but denture frameworks are lighter.
Fusion temperature	As high as 1500°C	Normally lower than 1000°C	Co/Cr alloys require electrical induction furnace or oxyacetylene equipment. Cannot use gypsum-bonded investments for Co/Cr alloys.
Tensile strength (MPa)	850	750	Both acceptable.
Proportional limit (MPa)	700	500	Both acceptable. Can resist stresses without deformation.
Modulus of elasticity (GPa)	220	100	Co/Cr more rigid for equivalent thickness. Advantage for connectors. Disadvantage for clasps.
Hardness (Vickers)	420	250	Co/Cr more difficult to polish but retains polish during service.
Ductility (percentage elongation)	2	15 (as cast) 8 (hardened)	Co/Cr clasps may fracture if adjustments are attempted.

Note: Values for gold alloy are for heat-hardened material except where indicated.

Table 8.2 Comparative properties of Ni/Cr alloys and type III casting gold alloys for small cast restorations

Property (units)	Ni/Cr	Type III gold alloy	Comments
Density (g/cm^3)	8	15	More difficult to produce defect-free castings for Ni/Cr alloys.
Fusion temperature	As high as 1350°C	Normally lower than 1000°C	Ni/Cr alloys require electrical induction furnace or oxyacetylene equipment.
Tensile strength (MPa)	600	540	Both adequate for the applications being considered.
Proportional limit (MPa)	230	290	Both high enough to prevent distortions for applications being considered. Note that values are lower than for partial denture alloys (Table 8.1).
Modulus of elasticity (GPa)	220	85	Higher modulus of Ni/Cr is an advantage for larger restorations e.g. bridges and for porcelain-bonded restorations.
Hardness (Vickers)	300	150	Ni/Cr more difficult to polish but retains polish during service.
Ductility (percentage elongation)	Up to 30%	20 (as cast) 10 (hardened)	Relatively large values suggest that burnishing is possible. However, large proportional limit values suggest high forces would be required.

8.5 **Comparison with casting gold alloys**

The properties of the two main groups of base metal casting alloys dictate that the Co/Cr alloys are primarily used for partial denture castings, where the high values of modulus of elasticity and proportional limit are of major importance whilst the Ni/Cr alloys are primarily used for small castings such as crowns and bridges. These two groups of base metal alloys offer alternatives to the casting gold alloys at potentially considerable savings in cost. Table 8.1 gives comparative properties of the Co/Cr alloys and the type IV casting gold alloys. Table 8.2 gives comparative properties of the Ni/Cr alloys and type III casting gold alloys.

Cast partial denture alloys

The two major components of cast partial denture frameworks are the connectors and clasps. The connectors should be rigid (high value of modulus of elasticity required) and should not be permanently deformed by the action of mechanical stresses (high value of proportional limit required). It can be seen from Table 8.1 that the Co/Cr alloys most closely meet these two requirements. For clasps, a high value of proportional limit is required in order to prevent deformation. A lower value of modulus of elasticity would enable the clasp to engage relatively deep undercuts due to its increased flexibility. In addition, the alloy used to construct clasps should ideally be ductile so that adjustments can be made to clasps without fracturing. The gold alloys most closely match the requirements for clasps since they have adequately

high proportional limits, lower values of modulus of elasticity than Co/Cr alloys and greater ductility.

In practice, connectors and clasps are generally cast together from the same alloy. For reasons of cost, Co/Cr alloys are almost universally used despite their limitations. When designing partial denture frameworks due regard must be paid to the high modulus values and low ductility of the Co/Cr alloys. Clasps should not be designed to engage deep undercuts and alterations by bending may result in fractures. A reduction in thickness of the Co/Cr alloy decreases the force necessary to push the clasp over the bulge of the tooth but leaves the clasp arm exposed to the dangers of deformation during cleaning and handling of the denture. By a reduction of the undercut to approximately half that engaged by a gold clasp, coupled with the use of a slightly thinner cross-section, a clasp of moderate retention and adequate functional life can be designed. The use of very small undercuts, however, requires precise positioning of the clasp arm and this is not always easy to achieve. Consequently, it is often found that Co/Cr clasps are either too retentive initially and slowly lose this retention due to permanent deformation or, alternatively, clasps may engage undercuts which are too small and give barely adequate retention.

The best of both worlds is to use Co/Cr alloy for the connectors and class IV gold alloy for clasps. Whilst it is possible to solder these structures together, corrosion at the joint is not uncommon and, where possible, the gold clasp should be attached to the denture via the polymeric denture base material.

Crown and bridge alloys

Alloys used for crown and bridge work should be hard, rigid and durable. Both Ni/Cr and gold alloys have adequate mechanical properties with the greater rigidity of the Ni/Cr alloys being an advantage for bridges, particularly those with large spans.

The success of crown and bridge alloys depends to a great extent on the accuracy with which the restorations can be cast. The gold alloys have a significant advantage from this point of view. They have greater density which results in better castability due to the high thrust which is generated by the alloy as it enters the mould. The gold alloys undergo less casting shrinkage (approximately 1·5 percent) when compared with the Ni/Cr alloys (2·3 percent). In the case of gold alloys, the shrinkage is well compensated for by dimensional changes in the investment mould. For Ni/Cr alloys the contraction is probably not as well compensated. This, occasionally, results in ill-fitting castings. One advantage of the Ni/Cr alloys, which results from their great hardness, is that the margins of the cast restoration are unlikely to be destroyed during polishing.

The Ni/Cr alloys are rarely used for all-metal cast restorations but are widely used in bonded porcelain or ceramometallic restorations (see p.74).

8.6 **Biocompatibility**

Base metal casting alloys contain some components which should be regarded as either toxic or known to cause allergic reactions in some people.

Beryllium is a known animal carcinogen and poses a potential threat to dental personnel who inhale metal dust during polishing or grinding procedures. It is essential that areas in which such operations are carried out are kept well ventilated. Some base metal alloys do not contain beryllium — a trend which is likely to increase as the toxic effects of this metal are subjected to greater scrutiny.

For the patient, the most immediate biocompatibility risk concerns nickel and the risk of allergic contact dermatitis. It is known that nickel causes more contact dermatitis than all other metals combined and that relatively small nickel concentrations can be problemmatical. Nickel-free base metal alloys are now available and are likely to gain fairly wide use as alternatives for those patients with known or suspected nickel allergy.

Titanium metal and alloys of titanium with other metals, for example vanadium, have excellent biocompatibility and are likely to be used more frequently for dental applications in the future.

9 Casting

9.1 Introduction

Previous chapters have dealt with wax-pattern materials, investment materials and casting alloys. This chapter describes how the investment mould is formed and how the wax pattern is replaced by the alloy using a casting process. One of several methods can be used for casting depending upon the alloy which is to be used.

There are several faults which can occur in alloy castings, most of which can be traced to incorrect selection of materials or faulty technique.

9.2 Investment mould

The various components of a typical investment mould are illustrated in Fig. 9.1.

The mould cavity is formed by allowing the investment to set around the wax pattern and associated sprue former and sprue base (crucible). After allowing the investment material to set, the sprue base and former are removed and the wax pattern 'burnt out' to leave the completed mould cavity. The choice of investment material depends on the type of alloy which is to be cast. The casting ring liner serves a dual purpose. It forms a relatively pliable lining to the inner surface of the rigid metal casting ring. This allows almost unrestricted setting expansion and thermal expansion of the investment. In addition, its thermal insulating properties ensure that the investment mould does not cool rapidly and contract after removal from the 'burn out' oven.

The temperature to which the investment mould is heated during 'burn out' deserves special mention since this controls the thermal expansion of the investment. For gold alloys, either a slow 'burn out' at 450°C or a more rapid 'burn out' at 700°C is commonly used with gypsum-bonded investments. For Ni/Cr alloys a temperature in the range 700−900°C is normal, whilst for Co/Cr alloys a 'burn out' temperature of 1000°C is typical.

Factors such as the length and diameter of the sprue and the distance of the mould cavity from the base of the mould all have an effect on the quality of the casting. For large castings, two or more sprues may be necessary in order to ensure that molten alloy is able to reach all parts of the mould cavity before solidifying.

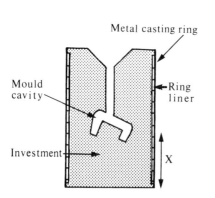

Fig. 9.1 Diagram illustrating components of an investment mould.

9.3 Casting machines

Numerous types of casting machines are available, the aim of each being to cause molten alloy to completely fill the investment mould cavity. The three main variables which characterize the machines are:

(1) The alloy may be melted in the mould sprue base (mould crucible) or in a separate crucible located in the casting machine,

(2) The alloy may be melted by one of several methods including gas−air torch, oxyacetylene torch, electrical induction heating or electrical resistance melting,

(3) The molten alloy may be driven into the mould by gravity, air pressure, steam pressure or

by centrifugal force. The arm of the centrifugal casting machine is rotated either by a spring or by means of an electric motor.

Possibly the most popular system in current use is that in which the alloy is melted in a separate crucible using electrical induction heating and forced into the mould using centrifugal force.

The classical approach to centrifugal casting was to have the casting ring attached to a chain. The alloy was melted in the mould sprue base and forced into the mould cavity by swinging the casting ring around at the end of the chain.

9.4 Faults in castings

The faults which can occur in castings may be of four types as follows:
  (1) Finning,
  (2) Incomplete casting,
  (3) Porosity in casting,
  (4) Oversized or undersized casting.

Finning Finning occurs when the investment is heated up too rapidly in the furnace. This causes the investment to crack. Molten alloy flows into the cracks forming thin 'fins' on the casting in regions where the cracks have been located.

Incomplete castings There are many possible causes of incomplete castings. In any casting the greater the number and thickness of the sprues, the more readily the metal will fill the mould. Against this, the sprues must be severed from the completed casting and an excessive number of sprues creates more work in finishing. Also, a larger weight of alloy is required for the casting and this presents difficulties in melting. It will be seen that the point of attachment of the sprues is a common site for defects and therefore an excessive number should be avoided.

If the alloy is not properly melted, or if the mould temperature is too low, solidification occurs before the mould can be properly filled. If there is insufficient thrust created during casting the alloy may not flow to all parts of the mould cavity. For centrifugal casting machines the thrust depends on the rotational speed of the casting arm, the length of the arm and the density of the alloy. The problem is therefore more significant for base metal alloys which have lower density and create less thrust.

Back pressure effects are caused by an inability of air or other gases within the mould to escape,

making way for the alloy. To assist the escape of gases, the investment material between the casting and the end of the ring should be as thin as is consistent with strength, (distance X in Fig. 9.1). Also, the end of the ring should not be completely covered by any part of the casting apparatus. In all cases the plate of metal which supports the end of the ring must be perforated.

Permeability of investments varies with particle size distribution, but generally it decreases in the order of gypsum-, phosphate- and silica-bonded. A rather dense layer of investment material is often created at the base of the ring, particularly when the base of the ring has been closed temporarily by a sheet of metal or glass. This dense layer should be scraped away to facilitate the escape of gases. When using silica-bonded or fine-grained, phosphate-bonded investments a vent, 0·5 mm in diameter, should be provided to allow escape of gases towards the crucible end of the mould. A casting which has been subjected to back pressure is rounded at the edges and lacking in detail.

Defects may also be caused by cooling shrinkage. On solidification, the alloy contracts but the outer portions of the casting remain in contact with the internal walls of the mould.

The thinner sections, or those portions which are less effectively insulated against heat loss by the investment material, freeze first. As they solidify they contract and draw molten metal from the remaining portions. Voids or secondary pipe will be formed unless more metal can enter the mould. Local shrinkage defects are commonly seen in the casting at the base of the sprue (Fig. 9.2). It is preferable, therefore, that the casting should freeze by a wave of solidification traversing its mass, moving towards the sprue. A reservoir of metal is

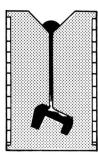

Fig. 9.2 Diagram illustrating a casting fault occurring at the base of the sprue.

then present within the sprues if these are of sufficient thickness. One method is to thicken up a section of each sprue as near to the casting as possible. These round *sprue reservoirs* should freeze last of all and any shrinkage porosity will be found in them, and not in the casting.

Porosity Porosity may be seen as surface pitting on the casting or may be revealed within the cast metal on filing and polishing. Broken pieces of investment, or particles of dirt which have fallen down the sprue, may become embedded in the casting and produce pitting of the surface. For this reason all casting moulds should be handled with the sprue downwards.

Gaseous porosity in castings is produced by gases which become dissolved in the molten alloy. Copper, gold, silver, platinum, and particularly palladium, all dissolve oxygen in the molten state. On cooling, the alloys liberate the adsorbed gases but some remains trapped when the alloy becomes rigid. This type of porosity may affect all parts of the casting. Its effects can be reduced by avoiding overheating of the alloy or casting in the atmosphere of an inert gas or vacuum.

Undersized or oversized castings The final 'fit' of a casting depends on a 'balancing out' of expansions and contractions which occur during its construction. The major dimensional changes involved are the casting shrinkage of the alloy which should be compensated for by the setting expansion, thermal expansion and 'inversion' of the investment. Faults in technique, for example, not heating the investment mould to a high enough temperature, may produce insufficient compensation for casting shrinkage.

It should be remembered, however, that other factors such as the choice of impression material and impression technique may also influence the final result.

10   Wrought Alloys

10.1 Introduction

The previous chapters have dealt with casting alloys and casting techniques. Casting, however, is not the only way in which metals can be shaped. An alternative approach is to use *cold working*, in which the metal is hammered, drawn or bent into shape at temperatures well below the recrystallization temperature of the metal, often at room temperature. Metal or alloy structures produced in this way are said to have a wrought structure and often rely for their special properties on the work hardening which takes place during shaping.

Examples of the use of wrought alloys in dentistry include materials for making instruments and burs, wires, and occasionally, denture bases. Steel and stainless steel are the most widely used wrought alloys and are therefore worthy of some detailed discussion.

10.2 Steel

Steel is an alloy of iron and carbon in which the carbon content is less than 2 percent. Greater quantities of carbon produce a very brittle alloy which is unsuitable for cold working. In the solid state, steel is able to adopt a variety of structures depending on the carbon content and temperature. Above 723°C an interstitial solid solution of carbon in a face-centred cubic iron matrix is formed. This solid solution, termed *austenite*, is unstable below 723°C (the *critical temperature*) and the face-centred cubic iron matrix breaks down to form two phases. One phase consists of a very dilute solid solution of carbon in iron (up to 0·02 percent C), called *ferrite*. The other phase is a specific compound of iron and carbon with formula Fe_3C, called *cementite*. The mixture of ferrite and cementite is termed *pearlite*. These transitions are illustrated in the iron−carbon phase diagram given in Fig. 10.1.

It can be seen that certain aspects of the iron−carbon phase diagram resemble that for a eutectic alloy shown in Fig. 6.10. The critical temperature (Tc) for the iron−carbon system is equivalent to the eutectic temperature which characterized the eutectic alloys. In both cases, the temperature in question indicates the point at which the alloys undergo phase separation. Eutectic refers to the behaviour of an alloy of two mutually insoluble metals during crystallization. In the case of the iron−carbon system the transitions occur within the solid state. An alloy containing 0·8 percent carbon (corresponding to point X in Fig. 10.1) is known as the eutectoid alloy. Alloys with greater concentrations of carbon are called *hypereutectoid* alloys and those with smaller carbon contents, *hypoeutectoid* alloys. Both hypereutectoid and hypoeutectoid alloys consist of a mixture of ferrite and cementite at room temperature. The hypereutectoid alloys contain relatively greater amounts of cementite whilst the hypoeutectoid alloys contain greater amounts of ferrite.

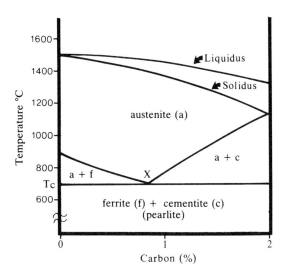

Fig. 10.1 The iron−carbon phase diagram (up to 2 percent carbon).

Cementite is a very hard, brittle material whilst ferrite is softer and more ductile. Hence the hypereutectoid steels which contain greater quantities of cementite are commonly used to produce cutting instruments such as burs. The hypoeutectoids are used for the construction of non-cutting instruments such as forceps.

Steel can be further hardened by heat treatment. If an alloy is heated to a temperature above the critical temperature but below the solidus temperature it forms an austenitic solid solution as shown in Fig. 10.1. If the alloy is then quenched there is insufficient time for the alloy to undergo the transition from the austenitic structure to the pearlite structure. Instead, a very hard and brittle steel, called *martensite*, which has a distorted body-centred cubic lattice, is formed. Martensite is too brittle for most applications but its brittleness can be reduced by using a low temperature heat treatment, called *tempering*. The alloy is heated to a

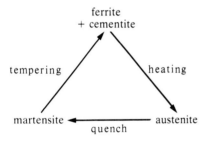

Fig. 10.2 Diagram illustrating the hardening and tempering cycle of heat treatments which can be used on steel.

temperature in the range 200–400°C, at which martensite partially converts to ferrite and cementite. The degree of conversion depends on the tempering temperature and the tempering time. Thus, the hardness and brittleness can be controlled quite accurately by choosing suitable heat treatment conditions. The process of heat treatment hardening and tempering is illustrated in Fig. 10.2.

The ability to be hardened by heat treatments is one of the major advantages of steel. Probably its main disadvantage is its susceptibility to corrosion.

10.3 Stainless steel
In addition to iron and carbon the stainless steels

contain chromium which improves corrosion resistance. This is achieved by the *passivating effect* in which the chromium exposed at the surface of the alloy is readily oxidized to form a tenacious surface film of chromic oxide. This film resists further attack from aqueous media thus preventing corrosion. Nickel is also present in many stainless steels. It contributes towards corrosion resistance and helps to strengthen the alloy.

The addition of chromium and nickel to steel causes the critical temperature (Tc) (see Fig. 10.1) to be lowered. If sufficient quantities of these two metals are incorporated, the austenitic structure remains even at room temperature. One of the most commonly used stainless steels contains 18 percent chromium and 8 percent nickel (termed *18/8 stainless steel*). This alloy has a critical temperature below room temperature and is therefore sometimes referred to as *austenitic stainless steel*. It is not possible to harden these stainless steels by heat treatment because the solid–solid transitions occur below room temperature. Hence, 18/8 stainless steels are used in applications where heat hardening is not necessary, for example, for non-cutting instruments, wires and occasionally as denture bases. These applications involve a degree of *cold working* since the alloy is shaped by either bending, drawing or swaging, all of which result in the formation of a wrought structure.

The method used for forming a stainless steel denture base deserves special mention. A thin sheet of 18/8 stainless steel (approximately 0·2 mm thick) is pressed between an alloy or epoxy resin die and counter die. The method of applying the pressure required for *swaging* may vary. Traditionally, a hydraulic press was used but modern techniques involve the use of a sudden pressure wave which adapts the sheet of alloy to the die very quickly. The pressure wave may be generated by using a controlled explosion or a sudden, controlled release of hydraulic pressure. These techniques are known as explosion forming and hydraulic forming respectively.

The advantages of the stainless steel denture base are that the base is thin, light and conducts heat rapidly, thereby ensuring that the patient retains a normal reflex reaction to hot and cold stimuli. The base is strong and has a good resistance to corrosion. The main disadvantages are the lack of surface detail on the swaged plate, and perhaps more significantly, the involved and time-consuming technique required for swaging, attaching retention tags by welding and processing of the acrylic parts of the denture.

When smaller quantities of chromium and nickel are incorporated into steel it is possible to produce an alloy which has adequate corrosion resistance but which can be hardened by heat treatment. An alloy with these characteristics may, typically, contain about 12 percent chromium and little or no nickel. This alloy is capable of forming a martensitic structure and is therefore sometimes referred to as *martensitic stainless steel*. This type of alloy is commonly used to construct cutting instruments and probes which can be hardened by heat treatment, using a technique similar to that previously described for steel.

10.4 Wires

Wires are commonly used for the construction of orthodontic appliances and occasionally as wrought clasps and rests on partial dentures. Wires are normally produced by drawing an ingot of alloy through dies of gradually decreasing cross-section to produce a circular, ovoid or square section wire in which the grain structure is highly fibrous in nature. (See p.45).

Requirements

The requirements of wires relate to their springiness, stiffness, ability to be bent without fracturing, corrosion resistance and an ability to be simply joined by soldering or welding. The springiness of a wire is a function of its fibrous grain structure which is incorporated during drawing of the wire. The 'springback' ability of a wire is a measure of its ability to undergo large deflections without permanent deformation. In terms of mechanical properties this is given by the ratio of yield stress to modulus of elasticity as follows:

$$\text{Springback potential} = \frac{\text{Yield stress}}{\text{Modulus of elasticity}}$$

A more approximate form of this equation uses proportional limit in place of yield stress.

A wire should have a value of stiffness, as indicated by its modulus of elasticity, which enables it to apply a suitable force for tooth movement during orthodontic treatment. This requirement varies considerably, since it is sometimes necessary to carry out rapid movements using stiff wires, whilst on other occasions it is necessary to apply small

forces with flexible wires in order to bring about slow movements.

Orthodontic wires are generally shaped by bending and the wire should possess sufficient ductility to resist fracture during this bending procedure.

Wires often remain in the oral cavity for several months, whether they be part of a fixed or a removable orthodontic appliance. The wire should therefore have good corrosion resistance in order that it can withstand attack from oral fluids.

Finally, it is sometimes necessary to join two parts of an appliance together and, ideally, wires should be capable of being easily joined either by soldering or by welding, without impairing the mechanical properties of the wire or reducing the corrosion resistance. The importance of this property is reduced in alloys which can be easily bent into loops as a means of joining.

Available materials

Table 10.1 lists the commonly used wires and summarizes their main properties.

Stainless steel   Stainless steel wires are constructed from the 18/8 austenitic type of stainless steel. They have a high value of modulus compared with some other alloys used to construct wires and are therefore used to apply relatively high forces. Lower forces can be achieved by using a wire of smaller diameter. 18/8 stainless steel has a relatively high value of yield stress and the 'springback' properties are thus adequate for most applications.

Stainless steel wires have sufficient ductility to allow bending without fracture. They can be obtained in three grades, often referred to as soft, half-hard and hard, ranging from very ductile (soft) to less ductile (hard). The type of wire is chosen according to the amount of bending which must be carried out. Following bending, a stress relief anneal can be carried out in order to relieve internal stresses. This involves heating the wire to 450°C for about ten minutes. The annealing procedure should be carried out only with 'stabilized' stainless steel wires which contain small quantities of titanium. Unstabilized wires become brittle during annealing due to a reaction between chromium and carbon.

Joining of stainless steel wires can be accomplished either by soldering or by welding. Silver solders are normally used for soldering. They contain silver and copper with small quantities of other

Table 10.1 Summary of properties of commonly used wires

Material	Stiffness	'Springback' ability	Ductility	Ease of soldering or welding
Stainless steel	High	Good	Adequate	Reasonable
Gold alloy	Medium	Adequate	Adequate	Easy to solder
Co/Cr alloy	High	Adequate following heat treatment	Good in soft state	Difficult
Ni/Ti alloy	Low	Excellent	Poor	Difficult
β-Ti	Medium	Good	Adequate	Joined by welding

elements to lower the fusion temperature. Care must be taken during soldering not to overheat the wires since this may cause recrystallization of the grain structure with a subsequent lack of springiness. In addition, overheating may cause the chromium to react with carbon, forming carbides, a phenomenon referred to as *weld decay*. This results in a loss of corrosion resistance around the soldered joint and the introduction of a degree of brittleness. The solder itself, of course, is a source of potential corrosion being of a eutectic-type composition.

Welding is accomplished by pressing two pieces of wire together between two electrodes then passing an electric current, sufficient to melt the wires at the point of contact joining them together. The temperature rise ($\triangle T$) at the joint when a current passes is given by the function,

$$\triangle T = \int (I^2 Rt)$$

where I is the current passing, R is the electrical resistence at the juntion of the two wires and t is the time for which the current passes.

High temperatures, sufficient for welding, can only be achieved with alloys giving relatively high values of electrical resistance at the junction. Thus, welding is not a suitable technique for joining gold wires. The electrical current and the time for which the current flows must be controlled such that adequate welding is achieved without overheating the rest of the wire. This would lead to weld decay and a degree of recrystallization, causing loss of the fibrous grain structure.

Gold alloys   The composition of gold alloy wires is similar to that of the type IV casting gold. A typical material contains 60 percent gold, 15 percent silver, 15 percent copper and about 10 percent platinum or palladium. The high platinum or palladium content raises the melting point and recrystallization temperature of the wires making them more amenable to soldering operations. Gold alloy wires have a lower value of modulus of elasticity than the stainless steel variety and therefore apply lower forces. An advantage of the gold alloy wires is that they are easily soldered using normal gold solders.

Cobalt–chromium alloys (elgiloy)   These alloys contain cobalt, chromium, nickel, iron and molybdenum in approximate proportions $40:20:15:16:7$. They have the unique characteristic of being supplied in a softened state which has excellent ductility. Following bending, the wire can be hardened by heat treating at 480°C. The precipitation hardening that occurs introduces the required springback properties into the wire.

The modulus of elasticity of the wire is similar to that for stainless steel, indicating a similar performance in terms of tooth movement. These wires are difficult to join by soldering.

Nickel–titanium alloys (nitinol)   These alloys contain almost equal amounts of nickel and titanium with small quantities of other metals. They are flexible wires with low modulus values and are used to apply relatively low forces. The low modulus coupled with high yield stress indicates excellent springback properties and they are particularly useful for carrying out large tooth movements using low forces over a long period of time. Nitinol wires have limited ductility and are not easy to bend without fracturing. They are not amenable to joining operations such as soldering or welding.

β-*Titanium* These alloys consist mainly of titanium with some molybdenum. They are ductile, allowing good formability, and have springback characteristics similar to those of stainless steel. They have a lower modulus value than stainless steel and therefore apply lower forces, and they can be joined by welding.

Porcelain and Metal-bonded Porcelain

11.1 Introduction

Fused porcelain has long been used in the construction of works of art. It can be produced in almost every shade or tint and its translucency imparts a depth of colour unobtainable by other materials. Although the technique of porcelain fusing is exacting it can be initially moulded by hand as a paste and additions or alterations can be made at various stages of the work. It is not surprising, therefore, that dentistry has turned to porcelain for the production of artificial teeth, crowns and bridges.

11.2 Composition of porcelain

The compositions of the various types of porcelain are summarized in Table 11.1. It can be seen that there are considerable differences in composition between the dental porcelains and decorative porcelain. Indeed, the dental porcelains contain little or no clay and, possibly, would be more aptly described as dental glasses.

Kaolin is a hydrated aluminosilicate, $Al_2O_3 \cdot 2SiO_2 \cdot 2H_2O$. The set decorative porcelain is essentially a mixture of this with silica, bound together by a flux or binder such as feldspar which is a mixture of potassium and sodium aluminosilicates, $K_2O \cdot Al_2O_3 \cdot 6SiO_2$ and $Na_2O \cdot Al_2O_3 \cdot 6SiO_2$. Feldspar is the lowest fusing component and it is this which melts and flows during firing, uniting the other components in a solid mass. The fusion temperature of feldspar may be further reduced by adding to it other low-fusing fluxes such as borax.

Of the two types of dental porcelain, the high-fusing materials fuse in the range 1300–1400°C whilst the low-fusing materials fuse in the range 850–1100°C. The latter materials are by far the more commonly used products.

The powders supplied to the dentist or technician are not just mixtures of the various ingredients. During manufacture the constituents are mixed together and then fused to form a *frit*. This is broken up, often by dropping the hot material into cold water. It is then ground into a fine powder ready for use.

In the fusion process which takes place during manufacture the flux reacts with the outer layers of the grains of silica, kaolin or glass and partly combines them together. When the technician fuses the porcelain powder, during the production of a crown for example, he simply remelts the fluxes without causing any significant increase in reaction between the flux and the other components.

Porcelain powders are sometimes pigmented in order that natural tooth shades can be matched. The *pigments* used are normally metal oxides which are stable at the fusion temperature.

The use of uranium compounds in dental porcelains to simulate tooth fluorescence is now considered inadvisable. It is not only unnecessary but can give an unnatural appearance under ultraviolet light and, in addition, may create a potential health hazard.

A low-fusing, transparent glass may be used as a *glaze* over the completed body of the porcelain restoration. The glaze gives the crown an impervious, smooth surface and imparts greater translucency.

A smooth surface can be obtained without using a glaze. By careful control of the furnace temperature, the surface of the normal porcelain will flow and glaze with only a slight rounding of the contours of the restoration. Unfortunately, any overheating will cause gross distortions of the shape.

The porcelain powders are mixed with water to produce a plastic mass of material which can be moulded and carved before firing. To improve the working properties a *binder* such as sugar or starch is added to some powders.

11.3 Compaction and firing

The aqueous plastic mass of porcelain particles is

Table 11.1 Composition of porcelains

Material	Components (percentage)			
	Clay (kaolin)	Silica	Binder (feldspar)	Glasses
Decorative porcelain	50	25	25	0
High-fusing dental	4	15	80	0
Low-fusing dental	0	25	60	15

compacted as much as possible onto a platinum foil matrix. This reduces the size of the spaces between the particles and thus reduces firing shrinkage. Powders consisting of a mixture of particle sizes compact more easily than those with particles of one size only.

The moulded crown may be lightly vibrated, thus helping to settle the powder particles and bring excess water to the surface, where it is blotted by an absorbent cloth. Alternatively, the powder may be 'patted' with a spatula to achieve the same effect.

A well-compacted crown not only reduces firing shrinkage but also shows a regular contraction over its entire surface, thus maintaining the original form on a slightly reduced scale.

Following compaction, the next stage involves porcelain 'firing'. A porcelain furnace consists, essentially, of an electrically heated muffle with a pyrometer which indicates the temperature in that part of the muffle where the porcelain is placed.

If the freshly compacted, wet structure is placed in a hot furnace it will evolve steam rapidly and crumble or even explode. The normal procedure, therefore, is to dry the wet structure in a warm atmosphere before placing into the hot furnace.

At the elevated temperatures of the furnace, the starch or sugar binder ignites and the surface of the structure blackens. The door of the furnace is left slightly ajar during this stage to allow the products of combustion to escape. The furnace door is then closed and firing is completed. Shrinkage takes place as the fluxes bind the particles together causing a uniform inward contraction of the whole mass. Further additions of fresh material may be made at this stage before glazing. Whenever porcelain work is heated or cooled the process must be carried out slowly. Porcelain is a poor conductor of heat and is brittle. Rapid cooling would result in

cracking and loss of strength.

The accuracy of fit is maintained by building up the porcelain on a platinum foil which has been closely adapted to the die. The firing shrinkage which occurs does not therefore cause a great discrepancy in the accuracy of fit, since the shrinkage occurs inwards towards the platinum foil and the foil itself is not affected by firing. Before cementation, the platinum foil is removed from the inner surface of a crown to create about 25 μm of space for cementation. The use of porcelain for constructing inlays is a most exacting technique because, in this case, firing shrinkage has a direct effect on the fit of the inlay. For this reason the porcelain inlay is a very rare restoration.

11.4 Properties of porcelain

Aesthetically, porcelain is an almost perfect material for the replacement of missing tooth substance. It is available in a range of shades and at various levels of translucency such that a most life-like appearance can be achieved. The inner layer of the porcelain crown, for example, is normally constructed from a fairly opaque 'core' material. This is overlaid with a more translucent 'dentine' material with a final coating of translucent 'enamel' porcelain forming the outermost layer.

Porcelain is a very rigid, hard and brittle material whose strength is dependent on the presence of surface irregularities or internal voids and porosities. Fine-grained powders give more uniform surfaces than coarser grains, and firing at reduced pressures can reduce porosity. The formation of

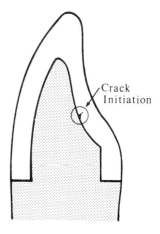

Fig. 11.1 Diagram illustrating the initiation and propagation of a crack from the inner surface of a porcelain crown.

superficial cracks due to thermal stresses are best avoided by slow cooling from the firing temperature. Fracture can be initiated from small surface scratches caused by grinding and these should be eliminated by smoothing or by further fusing. Cracks in porcelain crowns invariably emanate from the inner, unglazed fitting surface and propagate outwards towards the exposed surface material as illustrated in Fig. 11.1.

The relatively poor mechanical properties of porcelain can be improved using alumina, or metal supporting structures. These are discussed in the next sections.

Porcelain has excellent thermal properties and is a particularly good thermal insulator. This fact is of importance when gross amounts of enamel and dentine are to be replaced and the residual layer of dentine may be of minimal thickness.

Porcelain is very resistant to chemical attack, being unaffected by the wide variations of pH which may be encountered in the mouth.

11.5 Alumina inserts and aluminous porcelain

The major disadvantage of porcelain is brittleness and this is the factor which most limits its use. Several methods are available which are aimed at preventing the formation or propagation of cracks on the inner surface of porcelain restorations.

One approach is to use a core of pure alumina on which the porcelain crown is constructed. Alumina is a very hard, opaque material which is less susceptible to crack propagation than porcelain. The alumina core is often used in combination with a metal post which is inserted into the tooth following removal of the pulp. Another approach to

strengthening involves the use of pure alumina inserts. These may be in the form of small sheets of alumina which are generally placed palatally in a crown in order to strengthen without impairing the appearance.

Powdered alumina may be added to porcelain in order to achieve a significant strengthening. The mechanism of strengthening is that the alumina particles act as 'crack stoppers' preventing the propagation of a crack throughout the body of the porcelain (Fig. 11.2a). This improvement of properties is achieved not only as a result of the good mechanical properties of alumina but also due to the compatibility of alumina with porcelain. The two materials have closely matching values of coefficient of thermal expansion and modulus of elasticity. This ensures that the interface region between the alumina particles and the porcelain is virtually stress-free and not likely to encourage crack propagation around the alumina particles. Attempts to improve the properties of porcelain with materials which are not compatible have been unsuccessful since the cracks propagate around the 'reinforcing' material as illustrated in Fig. 11.2b.

Porcelain which contains alumina is referred to as aluminous porcelain and the alumina content is normally around 40 percent. Although aluminous porcelain has definite advantages in terms of mechanical properties, it is opaque and therefore can only be used to construct the inner core region of a porcelain crown. This is generally acceptable, since it is the inner region from which cracks propagate and which is therefore the area in need of reinforcement.

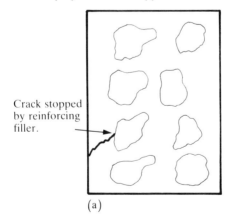

Crack stopped by reinforcing filler.

(a)

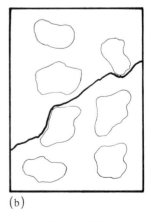

(b)

Fig. 11.2 Diagram illustrating how the propagation of a crack can be halted by a reinforcing particle. (a) Alumina particle acting as a crack stopper. (b) A crack propagating around a filler particle.

11.6 Metal-bonded porcelain

The metal-bonded porcelain restoration involves a marrying of the good mechanical properties of cast dental alloys with the excellent aesthetic properties of porcelain. Generally, the restorations consist of an alloy substructure with bonded porcelain veneers as shown in Fig. 11.3.

The requirements of the alloy used to form the substructure are similar to those for non-porcelain bonding work with additional requirements as follows:

(1) The alloy, having been previously cast into the desired shape, should be capable of withstanding porcelain firing without melting or suffering creep. Hence the alloy must have a high fusion temperature,

(2) The alloy should be sufficiently rigid to support a very brittle porcelain veneer otherwise fracture of the veneer is inevitable,

(3) The alloy should be capable of forming a bond with the porcelain veneer in order that the latter does not become detached,

(4) The alloy should have a value of coefficient of thermal expansion similar to that for the porcelain to which it is bonded.

There are four types of alloy currently available for porcelain bonding. These are (a) high-gold alloys, (b) low gold-content alloys, (c) silver–palladium alloys and (d) nickel–chromium alloys. Table 11.2 gives a summary of the comparative properties of the four alloys.

High-gold alloys

The composition of a typical high gold-content porcelain-bonding alloy is shown in Table 11.3. The major differences between these alloys and the non porcelain-bonding alloys are the high platinum/palladium content, the absence of copper and the presence of small amounts of base metals such as tin and indium.

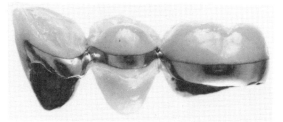

Fig. 11.3 Photograph showing a metal-bonded porcelain restoration. Porcelain veneers are built up on an alloy substructure.

The high platinum/palladium content raises the melting temperature of the alloy, reducing the risk of softening and creep during porcelain firing. In addition, these two metals decrease the coefficient of thermal expansion of the gold alloy to a value closer to that for porcelain. Copper is absent from porcelain-bonding gold alloys since, when present, it imparts a green hue to the porcelain veneer. The minor quantities of base metals such as tin and indium are essential in promoting bonding between the alloy and the overlying veneer. The base metals become oxidized at the surface and the oxide layer forms a chemical bond with porcelain during firing.

The high-gold alloys have two disadvantages when used for porcelain bonding. Despite the high platinum/palladium content, the melting range is still sufficiently low that there is a risk of alloy 'sag' during porcelain firing. Secondly, the modulus of elasticity of the high-gold alloys is less than ideal. Subsequently, *copings* must be produced in fairly thick section in order to prevent flexing which would result in porcelain fracture. The requirement of a minimum coping thickness of around 0·5 mm results in the risk of an over-contoured restoration and gingival irritation.

Low-gold alloys

Low-gold porcelain-bonding alloys contain approxi-

Table 11.2 Properties of alloys used for porcelain bonding

Alloy	Castability	Creep resistance during firing	Modulus	Bond strength	Biocompatibility
High-gold	+++	−	+	+	++
Low-gold	++	+	++	+	+
Silver–palladium	−	+	++	+	+
Nickel–chromium	−−	++	+++	−	−−−

Key +++ Excellent → −−− Poor

Table 11.3 Composition of a typical high gold-content
porcelain-bonding alloy

Metal	Percentage
Gold	85
Platinum	10
Palladium	3
Silver	1
Tin	0·5
Indium	0·5

mately 50 percent gold, 30 percent palladium to
raise the melting temperature and lower the coefficient of thermal expansion, 10 percent silver and 10
percent indium and tin for porcelain bonding.

The mechanical properties of the low-gold alloys
are similar to those for the high-gold materials.
They have a slightly greater modulus of elasticity
which is an advantage for porcelain bonding. The
higher melting range produces better creep resistance for these materials during porcelain firing.

Good properties and a significant cost saving
compared with high-gold alloys account for the
widespread use of these materials for bonded porcelain work.

Silver–palladium alloys
These alloys contain about 60 percent palladium,
30 percent silver and 10 percent indium and/or tin
to aid porcelain bonding. They have the advantages
of a higher modulus value and a higher melting
range than the high-gold alloys. They offer a suit-

able alternative to the high-gold materials for
bonded porcelain work at a considerable saving in
cost, providing care is taken during casting to avoid
defects and gas inclusions.

Nickel–chromium alloys
Nickel–chromium casting alloys typically contain
70–80 percent nickel and 10–25 percent chromium
with small quantities of other metals such as molybdenum, tungsten and beryllium. Porcelain bonding is to the layer of chromic oxide which forms on
the surface of the alloy.

These alloys have the advantages of a very high
modulus and high melting temperature. Their disadvantages are:

(1) A high casting shrinkage which may affect
accuracy of fit if not fully compensated by the
investment,

(2) A tendency for poor castability, with voids in
the castings,

(3) A bond strength with porcelain which does
not compare with that achieved with the other
alloys.

Indeed, fractures in Ni/Cr–porcelain systems
invariably occur through the oxide layer whereas
fractures in the other systems generally occur
cohesively in the porcelain. In addition, these
alloys are suspect from the biocompatibility point
of view, as discussed on p.61.

11.7 Bonded platinum foil
A problem with the metal-bonded porcelain restoration is that a considerable thickness of tooth substance must be removed to allow space for the
metal coping and the porcelain veneer. An alternative approach, which does not produce such a
robust result but which may be adequate in some
circumstances, is to make a porcelain crown which
is bonded to a platinum foil.

The technique involves laying down two platinum foils on the working die as opposed to the
normal single foil (Fig. 11.4). The exposed surface
of the outer foil is then tin plated and the porcelain
crown constructed and fired on top of the tin-plated
surface. Porcelain bonds to the layer of tin oxide on
the tin-plated surface. The inner platinum foil is
removed prior to cementation of the crown whilst
one platinum foil remains bonded to the inner
surface of the crown. This foil helps to prevent
crack formation on the inner surface.

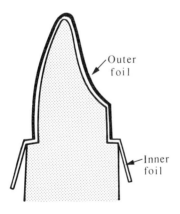

Fig. 11.4 Diagram illustrating two layers of closely
adapted platinum foil on a die prior to tin plating and
porcelain build-up.

12

Synthetic Polymers

12.1 Introduction

Synthetic polymers have been of importance for 60 years or more and find use in almost every sphere of modern life. Prior to the realization of the importance of such products they were often discarded as unwanted byproducts of other chemical processes.

Polymers are high molecular weight, chain-like molecules. A polymer chain does not consist of a random arrangement of atoms, but of distinct repeating groups of atoms, derived from the small molecules or *monomers* from which the chain is built up. The process by which monomers are converted into polymers is called polymerization.

Monomers are generally liquids or gases and during the process of polymerization they become converted to crystalline or amorphous solids. These may vary from being very rigid at one extreme to being soft and rubbery at the other.

12.2 Polymerization

The conversion of monomer molecules into polymers may proceed by either an *addition* reaction or a *condensation* reaction.

Addition polymerization

An addition reaction simply involves the joining together of two molecules to form a third, larger molecule. For example, ethylene reacts with bromine under the correct conditions to form dibromoethane, as follows:

$$CH_2{=}CH_2 + Br_2 \rightarrow CH_2Br{-}CH_2Br$$

Addition polymerizations involve the addition of a reactive species with a monomer to form a larger reactive species which is capable of further addition with monomer. In simplified terms the reaction may be visualized as follows:

$$R^* + M \rightarrow R - M^*$$
$$R - M^* + M \rightarrow R - M - M^*$$
$$R - M - M^* + M \rightarrow R - M - M - M^* \text{ etc.}$$

The initial reactive species is represented by R^* and the monomer molecules by M. It can be seen how monomer molecules are added during each stage of the polymerization reaction and eventually a long-chain molecule is produced.

The reactive species which is involved in the addition reaction may be ionic in nature or it may be a free radical. *Free radical addition polymerization* is very commonly used for the synthesis of polymers and is the method used in many dental polymers. The free radicals are produced by reactive agents called *initiators*. These are, generally, molecules which contain one relatively weak bond which is able to undergo decomposition to form two reactive species, each carrying an unpaired electron. One very popular initiator, which is used extensively in dental polymers, is benzoyl peroxide. Under certain conditions the peroxide linkage is able to split to form two identical radicals as shown in Fig. 12.1. The decomposition of benzoyl peroxide may be accomplished either by heating or by reaction with a chemical *activator*. The use of a chemical activator allows polymerization to occur at low temperatures. Activators commonly used with peroxide initiators are aromatic tertiary amines such as N, N'dimethyl-p-toluidine (Fig. 12.2).

An alternative activation system involves the use of radiation to cause decomposition of a suitable radiation-sensitive initiator. For example, benzoin methyl ether decomposes to form free radicals when exposed to ultraviolet radiation. Certain

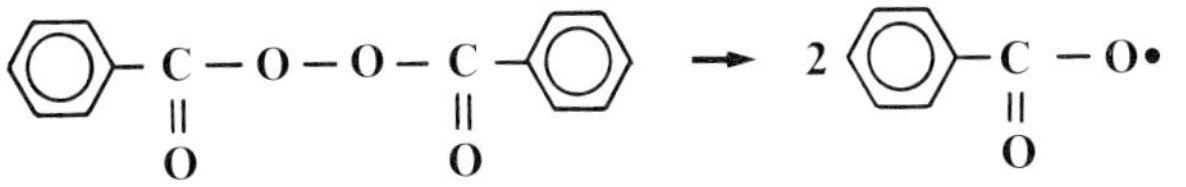

Fig. 12.1 Benzoyl peroxide readily splits to form two identical free radicals which can initiate polymerization.

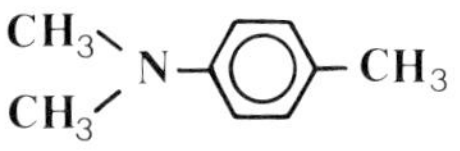

Fig. 12.2 *N, N'* dimethyl-*p*-toluidine — a tertiary amine which is capable of activating peroxide initiators.

ketones, when exposed to radiation in the visible spectrum range and in the presence of a tertiary amine, are capable of forming active radicals which can initiate polymerization.

The majority of monomers which can be polymerized by a free radical addition mechanism are of the alkene type. That is, they contain a carbon–carbon double bond. These monomers can be represented by the general formula given in Fig. 12.3. Some of the familiar monomers which can be obtained by substituting for X and Y in the figure are also given. Methylmethacrylate and other closely related monomers are of particular importance in dentistry.

The polymerization processes follows a well-documented pattern which consists of four main stages — *activation*, *initiation*, *propagation* and *termination*.

Activation This involves decomposition of the peroxide initiator using either thermal activation (heat), chemical activators or radiation of a suitable wavelength if a radiation-activated initiator is present. For benzoyl peroxide the activation reaction is represented by the equation given in Fig. 12.1 In simplified, general terms it may be expressed as follows:

$$R - O - O - R \rightarrow 2RO.$$

where R represents any organic molecular grouping.

Initiation The polymerization reaction is initiated when the radical, formed on activation, reacts with a monomer molecule. This is illustrated for the specific case of the benzoyl peroxide radical and the methacrylate monomer in Fig. 12.4. The reaction may be given in simplified general terms as follows:

$$RO \cdot + M \rightarrow RO - M \cdot$$

where the symbol M represents one molecule of monomer. It can be seen from the above equation and from Fig. 12.4 that the initiation reaction is an addition reaction producing another active free radical species which is capable of further reaction.

Propagation Following initiation, the new free radical is capable of reacting with further monomer molecules. Each stage of the reaction produces a new reactive species capable of further reaction, as illustrated in the following equations:

$$RO - M \cdot + M \rightarrow RO - M - M \cdot$$
$$RO - M - M \cdot + M \rightarrow RO - M - M - M \cdot$$
$$RO - M - M - M \cdot + M \rightarrow RO - M - M - M - M \cdot$$

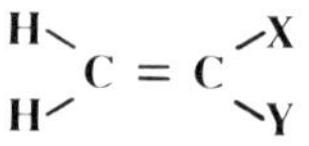

X	Y	Monomer	Polymer
H	H	Ethylene	Polyethylene
H	Cl	Vinyl chloride	Polyvinylchloride(PVC)
H	Phenyl	Styrene	Polystyrene
H	$-CH=CH_2$	Butadiene	Polybutadiene
H	$-CO_2CH_3$	Methylacrylate	Polymethylacrylate
CH_3	$-CO_2CH_3$	Methylmethacrylate	Polymethylmethacrylate

Fig. 12.3 General formula for alkene molecules which are capable of polymerizing to form polymers. Examples of some specific monomers are given.

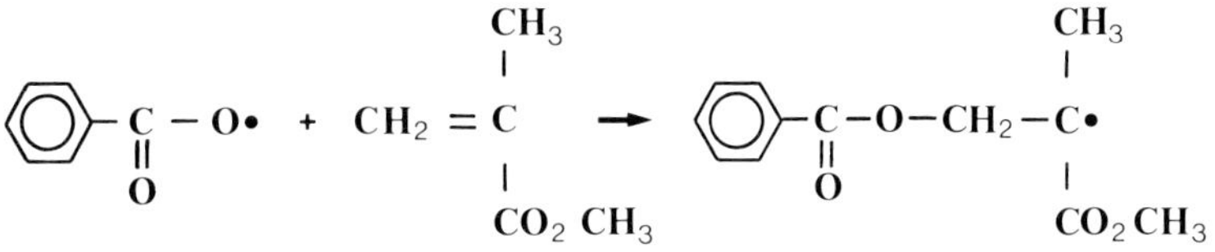

$$\bigcirc\!\!\!\!-\!\!\overset{\displaystyle \underset{\|}{\text{C}} - \text{O}\bullet}{\underset{\text{O}}{}} \quad + \quad \text{CH}_2 = \overset{\displaystyle \underset{|}{\text{CH}_3}}{\underset{\text{CO}_2\,\text{CH}_3}{\text{C}}} \quad \longrightarrow \quad \bigcirc\!\!\!\!-\!\!\overset{\displaystyle \underset{\|}{\text{C}} - \text{O} - \text{CH}_2 - \text{C}\bullet}{\underset{\text{O}}{}} \overset{\displaystyle \underset{|}{\text{CH}_3}}{\underset{\text{CO}_2\,\text{CH}_3}{}}$$

Fig. 12.4 The ·reaction of a benzoyl peroxide radical with methylmethacrylate to form a new radical species. This is the initiation reaction in free radical polymerization of methylmethacrylate.

A general equation for the propagation reaction may be written as follows:

$$RO - M\cdot + nM \rightarrow RO - (M)_n - M\cdot$$

where the value of n defines the number of monomer molecules added and hence the length of the chain and the molecular weight.

Termination It is possible for the propagation reaction to continue until the supply of monomer molecules is exhausted. In practice however, other reactions, which may result in the termination of a polymer chain, compete with the propagation reaction. These reactions produce 'dead' polymer chains which are not capable of further additions.

One example of termination is the combination of two growing chains to form one 'dead' chain as follows:

$$RO - (M)_n - M\cdot + RO - (M)_x - M\cdot \rightarrow$$
$$RO - (M)_n - M - M - (M)_x - OR$$

Other examples of termination involve the reactions of growing chains with molecules of initiator, 'dead' polymer, impurity or solvent, if present.

Factors which have an important influence on the properties of the resulting polymer are *molecular weight* and the degree of *chain branching* or *cross-linking*.

Molecular weight Within any addition polymerization system, activation, initiation, propagation and termination reactions occur simultaneously and the resulting polymer is therefore composed of chains of varying lengths. Thus, it is not possible to define a precise molecular weight for polymers and they are normally characterized in terms of an average molecular weight.

Chain branching and cross-linking Addition polymerization reactions generally lead to the production of *linear polymers*. This does not imply that the chains form straight lines but simply that there are no branches off the main polymer chain and that the chains are not linked together.

Chain branching may result if a growing chain undergoes *chain transfer* with a polymer molecule. This involves termination of the growing chain, but a new reactive radical is formed along the side of a polymer molecule. Growth of a fresh chain from this site produces a branched polymer. This is illustrated in Fig. 12.5.

Cross-linking is accomplished by adding *cross-linking agents* to the polymerizing monomer. In the case of free radical addition polymerizations these agents are invariably difunctional alkenes in which each of the two double bonds present is able to become polymerized into a separate chain, thus effectively linking two chains together. Fig. 12.6 shows the general formula for a typical cross-linking agent and the way in which this gives a cross-linked polymer when it becomes involved in a polymerization reaction. Fig. 12.7 gives the structural formula of ethylene glycol dimethacrylate, a cross-linking agent which is commonly used for methacrylate polymers.

Chain branching and cross-linking can have important effects on the properties of polymers.

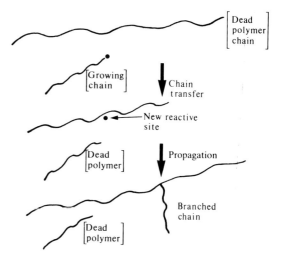

Fig. 12.5 Diagram showing the production of branched polymer chains by chain transfer.

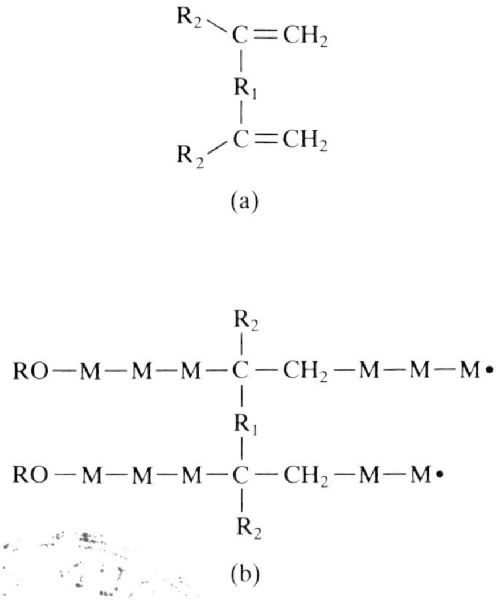

$$R_2 \diagdown C{=}CH_2$$
$$|$$
$$R_1$$
$$|$$
$$R_2 \diagup C{=}CH_2$$

(a)

$$R_2$$
$$|$$
$$RO-M-M-M-C-CH_2-M-M-M\bullet$$
$$|$$
$$R_1$$
$$|$$
$$RO-M-M-M-C-CH_2-M-M\bullet$$
$$|$$
$$R_2$$

(b)

Fig. 12.6 (a) General formula of a difunctional molecule which is capable of acting as a cross-linking agent. (b) The incorporation of the cross-linking agent into two polymer chains causes linking.

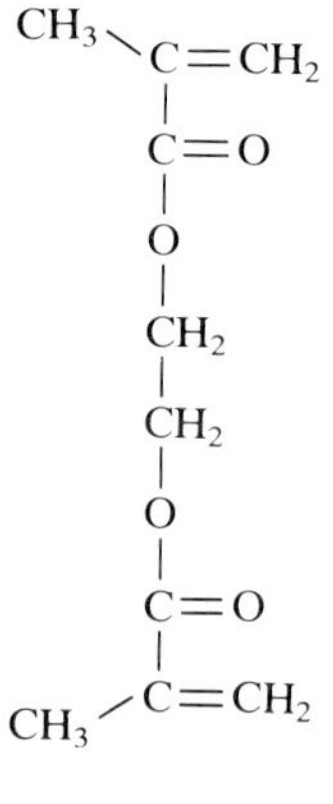

$$CH_3 \diagdown C{=}CH_2$$
$$|$$
$$C{=}O$$
$$|$$
$$O$$
$$|$$
$$CH_2$$
$$|$$
$$CH_2$$
$$|$$
$$O$$
$$|$$
$$C{=}O$$
$$|$$
$$CH_3 \diagup C{=}CH_2$$

Fig. 12.7 The structural formula of ethylene glycol dimethacrylate, a commonly used cross-linking agent.

Condensation polymerization

A condensation reaction involves two molecules reacting together to form a third, larger molecule with the production of a byproduct which is normally a small molecule such as water. A simple example of a condensation reaction is an esterification reaction in which an organic acid and an alcohol react together to form an ester with the evolution of water. This reaction may be illustrated by the reaction between acetic acid and ethyl alcohol to form ethyl acetate:

$$CH_3CO_2H + C_2H_5OH \rightarrow CH_3CO_2C_2H_5 + H_2O$$

A simple generalized reaction sequence for condensation polymerization for two monomers, $X{-}M_1{-}X$ and $Y{-}M_2{-}Y$, with reactive groups X and Y can be written as follows:

$$X - M_1 - X + Y - M_2 - Y \rightarrow$$
$$X - M_1 - M_2 - Y + XY$$
$$X - M_1 - M_2 - Y + X - M_1 - X \rightarrow$$
$$X - M_1 - M_2 - M_1 - X + XY$$
$$X - M_1 - M_2 - M_1 - X + Y - M_2 - Y \rightarrow$$
$$X - M_1 - M_2 - M_1 - M_2 - Y + XY \text{ etc.}$$

It can be seen that at each stage of the reaction the chain grows by one monomer unit and there is one molecule of byproduct XY evolved. In addition, the growing polymer chain retains two reactive groups at each stage. The resulting polymer is a regular copolymer of the monomers M_1 and M_2 which are arranged in sequence along the chain. Chain branching and cross-linking can be produced by introducing some trifunctional monomer

e.g.
$$X$$
$$|$$
$$X - M_1 - X$$

into the reaction.

By using a monomer which carries two reactive groups it is possible to produce a homopolymer as follows:

$$X - M_1 - Y + X - M_1 - Y \rightarrow$$
$$X - M_1 - M_1 - Y + XY$$
$$X - M_1 - M_1 - Y + X{-}M_1{-}Y \rightarrow$$
$$X - M_1 - M_1 - M_1 - Y + XY$$
$$X - M_1 - M_1 - M_1 - M_1 - Y + X - M_1 - Y \rightarrow$$
$$X - M_1 - M_1 - M_1 - M_1 - Y + XY \text{ etc.}$$

Examples of the use of condensation polymerization include the production of nylon 6,6 as illustrated in Fig. 12.8, the production of nylon 6, as illustrated in Fig. 12.9, and the synthesis of polydimethylsiloxane (silicone rubber) as illustrated in Fig. 12.10. The latter example illustrates the simplest type of condensation polymerization, in which each molecule contains two identical reactive groups (hydroxyl groups in this case) which are capable of reacting to eliminate water.

$$H_2N(CH_2)_6\ NH_2\ +\ HO_2C(CH_2)_4\ CO_2H$$

$$\swarrow -H_2O$$

$$H_2N(CH_2)_6\ NH\ CO(CH_2)_4\ CO_2H\ +\ H_2N(CH_2)_6\ NH_2$$

$$\swarrow -H_2O$$

$$H_2N(CH_2)_6\ NH\ CO(CH_2)_4\ CO\ NH(CH_2)_6\ NH_2\ +\ HO_2C(CH_2)_4\ CO_2H$$

$$\swarrow -H_2O$$

$$H_2N(CH_2)_6\ NH\ CO(CH_2)_4\ CO\ NH(CH_2)_6\ NH\ CO(CH_2)_4\ CO_2H$$

$$\swarrow$$

etc.

Fig. 12.8 Schematic representation of the condensation reaction between hexamethylene diamine and adipic acid to produce nylon 6,6.

$$H_2N\ (CH_2)_5\ CO_2H\ +\ H_2N\ (CH_2)_5\ CO_2H$$

$$\swarrow -H_2O$$

$$H_2N\ (CH_2)_5\ CO\ NH\ (CH_2)_5\ CO_2H\ +\ H_2N(CH_2)_5\ CO_2H$$

$$\swarrow -H_2O$$

$$H_2N\ (CH_2)_5\ CO\ NH\ (CH_2)_5\ CO\ NH\ (CH_2)_5\ CO_2\ +\ H_2N\ (CH_2)_5\ CO_2H$$

$$\swarrow -H_2O$$

$$H_2N(CH_2)_5\ CO\ NH(CH_2)_5\ CO\ NH(CH_2)_5\ CO\ NH(CH_2)_5\ CO_2H\quad etc.$$

Fig. 12.9 Schematic representation of the formation of nylon 6 by the condensation of hydrolysed caprolactam.

12.3 **Structure and properties**

Factors which control the structure and therefore the properties of polymers include:

(1) The molecular structure of the repeating units including the use of copolymers,

(2) The molecular weight or chain length,

(3) The degree of chain branching,

(4) The presence of cross-linking and the *cross-link density*,

(5) The presence of *plasticizers* or *fillers*.

Two basic properties which characterize polymers are *glass transition temperature* (Tg) and *melting temperature* (Tm). Crystalline polymers exhibit both a glass transition temperature and a melting temperature. Amorphous polymers, on the other hand, exhibit only a glass transition temperature. The latter materials are more widely used in dentistry. The glass transition temperature is the temperature at which molecular motions become such that whole chains are able to move. This tempera-

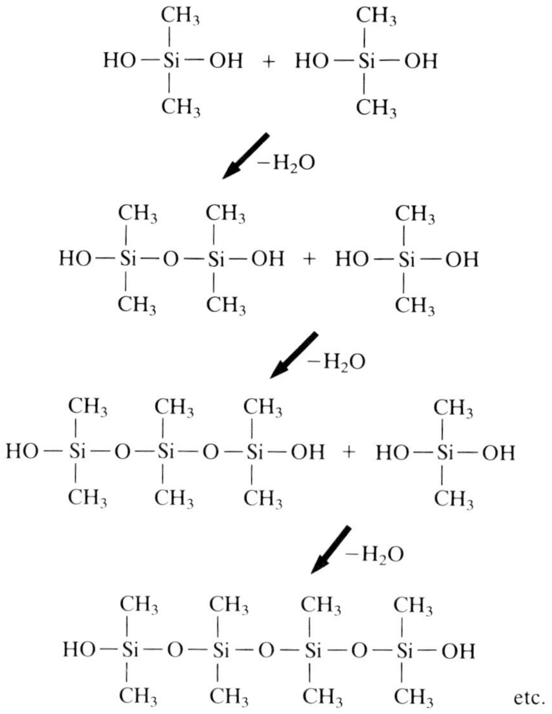

Fig. 12.10 The formation of hydroxyl-terminated polydimethylsiloxane by condensation of hydrolysed dimethylsiloxane.

ture is close to the 'softening temperature' which can be observed in practice for amorphous polymers. The glass transition temperature can be estimated mechanically by noting the temperature at which a sudden change in elastic modulus occurs.

Amorphous polymers below their glass transition temperature generally behave as rigid solids whilst above the glass transition temperature they may behave as viscous liquids, flexible solids or rubbers, depending on the molecular structure and the degree of branching or cross-linking.

From a practical point of view the value of Tg has great significance. For example, if a denture were constructed from a polymer which had a Tg value of 60°C, the denture would be rigid at normal mouth temperature but might soften and become flexible on taking a hot drink at 70°C.

Molecular structure is the factor which, naturally, has the greatest influence over polymer properties. For example, polymer backbones which contain phenyl groups are more rigid than those which contain only carbon–carbon bonds whilst backbones with silicon–oxygen bonds tend to be even more flexible. Hence the introduction of a phenyl group

into a polymer backbone has the effect of increasing Tg whilst the introduction of carbon–oxygen links has the reverse effect. It is not only the atomic groups forming the backbone of the polymer chain which have an effect on Tg. Pendant groups may have an equally marked effect. This is illustrated by considering the Tg values of a series of poly N-alkyl methacrylates where the alkyl group can be methyl, ethyl, propyl or butyl (Table 12.1). It can be seen that altering the pendent group in this series of polymers has a significant effect. Polymethylmethacrylate is rigid at mouth temperature whereas polybutylmethacrylate is relatively soft and flexible.

Table 12.1 Glass transition temperatures of N-alkyl methacrylate polymers

Polymer	Tg°C
Polymethylmethacrylate	105
Polyethylmethacrylate	65
Polypropylmethacrylate	35
Polybutylmethacrylate	20

Molecular weight is another factor which affects Tg. The two properties are related by an equation of the type

$$Tg = Tg_0 - \frac{K}{M}$$

where K is a constant, M is the average molecular weight and Tg_0 is the glass transition temperature for a polymer of infinite molecular weight. It can be seen that the value of Tg increases with increasing molecular weight. As M becomes large Tg approaches Tg_0. The reduction of the average molecular weight of a polymer by low molecular weight chains or residual, unreacted monomer may have a considerable effect on the Tg value and hence on material performance. In addition to influencing the glass transition temperature, molecular weight has an effect on other fundamental properties, such as modulus of elasticity. Many polymers exhibit a linear relationship between molecular weight and modulus up to fairly high values of molecular weight (10^5 or above) then reach a plateau region in which further increases in molecular weight have little or no effect.

Chain branching may have an effect on polymer properties. Increasing the concentration of branches generally lowers the glass transition temperature.

The effect of cross-linking is of considerable practical importance. Increasing the number of cross-links increases the glass transition temperature. In addition, alteration of the cross-link density can have a considerable effect on mechanical properties. A material with a low value of Tg and a small cross-link density may behave as a rubber at room temperature. On the other hand, a very high cross-link density normally produces a rigid, brittle polymer in which it is not possible to detect a glass transition since the material often decomposes thermally before softening. An example of this behaviour is the effect of cross-linking on the properties of natural rubber. When natural rubber (polyisoprene) is lightly cross-linked (vulcanized) it has rubbery, elastic properties. When the same material is highly cross-linked however, it becomes hard, rigid and brittle. This highly cross-linked material, vulcanite, has been used as a denture base material.

Certain additives such as plasticizers and fillers can have a profound effect on the properties of polymers. Plasticizers such as di-*n*-butylphthalate (Fig. 12.11) have an effect on both the glass transition temperature and the modulus of elasticity of some polymers. They are said to 'lubricate' the

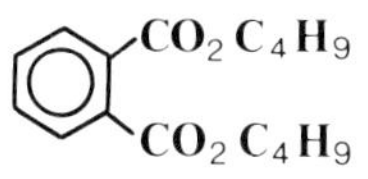

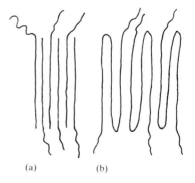

Fig. 12.11 Structural formula of di-*n*-butyl phthalate, a commonly used plasticizer.

movements of polymer chains, causing a lowering of Tg and a large decrease in elastic modulus. For this reason the inclusion of plasticizers is a common method used by manufacturers to produce 'soft' polymers.

The inclusion of particulate or fibrous inorganic fillers has an equally significant effect on polymer properties. The modulus of elasticity and strength are generally increased although, in the case of fibre-filled polymers, a degree of *anisotropy* may exist; that is, the strength depends on the orientation of the fibres in the polymer.

Particulate fillers are often used to increase the hardness of the resin and improve its resistance to abrasion. In addition, these fillers may have an important effect on thermal properties, since the added fillers are commonly glasses, ceramics or quartz which have lower values of coefficient of thermal expansion than organic polymers.

Crystalline polymers are normally formed when polymer chains are able to undergo orientation. Crystallites often take the form of polymer chains in rows, held together by Van der Waals forces or hydrogen bonds. The crystals may consist simply of straight chains or of folded chains as illustrated in Fig. 12.12. In order to form crystals of this type the chains must be able to come into close proximity with the neighbouring chain. Hence, the presence of bulky pendant groups and regular chain bran-

(a)   (b)

Fig. 12.12 Crystalline polymers may take one of several possible structural forms. Two examples are: (a) straight chains forming crystallites; (b) folded chains forming crystallites.

ching are factors which decrease the possibility of crystallite formation.

In nylon, the chains take up a helical form in which hydrogen bonding is responsible for both intramolecular and intermolecular links in the crystals.

Crystalline polymers have limited use in dentistry because they tend to be opaque and are not amenable to polymerization under ambient conditions of temperature and pressure.

12.4 Methods of fabricating polymers

Some polymers are produced in powder form and fabricated at a later stage by softening and moulding. Techniques for moulding include *injection moulding*, *vacuum forming* and *'blow' moulding*. Polymers which can be fabricated in this way are described as *'thermoplastic' polymers*, that is, they can be softened on heating and re-hardened on cooling. Providing care is taken not to overheat the polymer, causing decomposition, the process can be repeated many times.

Other polymers are described as *thermosetting*

resins — these are generally condensation polymers which are partly polymerized before moulding to produce a viscous liquid. During heating and moulding, generally into simple shapes such as flat sheets, the polymerization and cross-linking are completed. These resins are generally highly cross-linked polymers which cannot be softened without causing thermal degradation.

A method commonly used for dental polymers is to blend the monomer with an inert filler to form a paste. The paste is then split into two halves to which initiator and activator are added respectively. On mixing the two pastes the polymerization reaction begins and, for dental restorative materials, is completed *in situ*.

The technique of *dough moulding* is very important to dentistry, particularly for the fabrication of denture bases. Powdered polymer, normally as beads, containing some initiator is mixed with monomer to form a 'dough'. The dough is packed into a preformed mould and the monomer cured by applying heat. Alternatively, if the monomer contains a chemical activator the polymerization of monomer will occur at room temperature.

Denture Base Polymers

13.1 Introduction

The denture base is that part of the denture which rests on the soft tissues and so does not include the artificial teeth. Prior to 1940 vulcanite was the most widely used denture base polymer. This is a highly cross-linked natural rubber which was difficult to pigment and tended to become unhygienic due to the uptake of saliva. Nowadays acrylic resin is used almost universally for denture base construction.

The acrylic denture base is normally fabricated in a two-part gypsum mould. The mould is produced by investing wax trial dentures on which the artificial teeth have been mounted. After 'boiling out' of the wax the gypsum mould is treated with an alginate mould-sealing agent. This is a viscous solution of sodium alginate which is rapidly converted to calcium alginate on contact with the gypsum. It forms a thin 'skin' over the surface of the mould, preventing monomer in the acrylic 'dough' from entering the gypsum. The space remaining after removal of wax is filled with acrylic 'dough' which may be heat cured or allowed to cure at room temperature depending on the material being used. During curing the acrylic resin denture base becomes attached to the artificial teeth. The formation of the denture base by this technique is known as the *dough moulding method*. Acrylic denture bases may also be produced by *injection moulding* or by using a *pourable resin technique*, although the latter methods are not commonly used.

13.2 Requirements of denture base polymers

The requirements of a denture base material can be conveniently listed under the headings of physical, mechanical, chemical, biological and miscellaneous properties.

Physical properties An ideal denture base material should be capable of matching the *appearance* of the natural oral soft tissues. The importance of this requirement varies considerably, depending on whether the base will be visible when the patient opens his mouth.

A polymer which is used to construct a denture base should have a value of *glass transition temperature* (Tg) which is high enough to prevent softening and distortion during use. Although the normal temperature in the mouth varies only from 32°C to 37°C, account must be taken of the fact that patients take hot drinks at temperatures up to 70°C and, despite advice, sometimes clean dentures in very hot or even boiling water.

The base should have good *dimensional stability* in order that the shape of the denture does not change over a period of time. In addition to distortions which may occur due to thermal softening, other mechanisms such as relief of internal stresses, continued polymerization and water absorption may contribute to dimensional instability.

The material should, ideally, have a low value of *specific gravity* in order that dentures should be as 'light' as possible. This reduces the gravitational displacing forces which may act on an upper denture.

A high value of *thermal conductivity* would enable the denture wearer to maintain a healthy oral mucosa and to retain a normal reaction to hot and cold stimuli. If the base is a thermal insulator it is possible that the patient may take a drink which he would normally detect as being 'too hot to bear', and undergo a painful experience as the drink reaches the throat and gut.

The denture base should, ideally, be *radiopaque*. It should be capable of detection using normal diagnostic radiographic techniques. Patients occasionally swallow dentures and may even inhale fragments of dentures if involved in a violent accident, such as a car crash. Early radiological detection of the denture or fragment of denture is of immense help in deciding the best course of treatment.

Mechanical properties Although opinion varies slightly, most clinicians consider that the denture base should be rigid. A high value of *modulus of elasticity* is therefore advantageous. A high value of *elastic limit* is required to ensure that stresses encountered during biting and mastication do not cause permanent deformation. A combination of a high modulus and high value of elastic limit would have the added advantage that it would allow the base to be fabricated in relatively thin section.

Fractures of upper dentures invariably occur through the midline of the denture, due to flexing (Fig. 13.1). The denture base should have sufficient *flexural strength* to resist fracture. The method of measuring flexural strength or transverse strength is described on p.7.

Fracture of the denture base *in situ* often occurs by a fatigue mechanism in which relatively small flexural stresses, over a period of time, eventually lead to the formation of a small crack which propagates through the denture, resulting in fracture. The base material should therefore have an adequate *fatigue life* and a high value of *fatigue limit*.

When patients remove dentures for cleaning or overnight soaking, there is a danger of fracture if the denture is accidentally dropped onto a hard surface. The ability of a denture base to resist such fracture is a function of the *impact strength* of the material. Impact fracture of the denture may occur *in situ* if the patient is involved in a violent accident involving the facial region, for example, if the head hits a windscreen during a motor accident. The fragments of denture may then become embedded into soft tissue or inhaled.

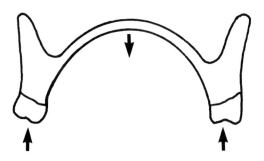

Fig. 13.1 Diagram illustrating how an upper denture may flex about the midpoint of the palate. This fatigue process may eventually cause fracture.

Denture base materials should have sufficient *abrasion resistance* to prevent excessive wear of material by abrasive denture cleansers or foodstuffs. Wear is a complex phenomenon which may depend on many material properties. For abrasive wear it is thought that surface hardness of the substrate is of primary importance.

Chemical properties A denture base material should be chemically inert. It should, naturally, be insoluble in oral fluids and should not absorb water or saliva since this may alter the mechanical properties of the material and cause the denture to become unhygienic.

Biological properties In the unmixed or uncured states the denture base material should not be harmful to the technician involved in its handling. The 'set' denture base material should be non-toxic and non-irritant to the patient. In the previous section it was mentioned that the base should, ideally, be impermeable to oral fluids and this would certainly be an ideal property. If a degree of absorption occurs however, the base should not be able to sustain the growth of bacteria or fungi.

Miscellaneous properties An ideal denture base material should be relatively inexpensive and have a long shelf life so that material can be purchased in bulk and stored without deteriorating. The material should be easy to manipulate and fabricate without having to resort to using expensive processing equipment. If fractures do occur they should be easy to repair.

13.3 Acrylic denture base materials
Acrylic resin is the most widely used material for construction of dentures.

Composition
The materials are normally supplied as a powder and liquid, details of the composition of which are given in Table 13.1. The major component of the powder is beads of polymethylmethacrylate with diameters up to 100 μm. These are produced by a process of *suspension polymerization* in which methylmethacrylate monomer, containing initiator, is suspended as droplets in a solution of starch or carboxymethylcellulose. The temperature is raised in order to decompose the peroxide and bring

Table 13.1 Composition of acrylic denture base materials

Powder	Polymer	Polymethylmethacrylate beads.
	Initiator	A peroxide such as benzoyl peroxide (approximately 0·5 percent).
	Pigments	Salts of cadmium or iron or organic dyes.
Liquid	Monomer	Methylmethacrylate.
	Cross-linking agent	Ethyleneglycoldimethacrylate (approximately 10 percent).
	Inhibitor	Hydroquinone (trace).
	Activator*	N, N'-dimethyl-p-toluidine (approximately 1 percent).

*Only in self-curing materials.

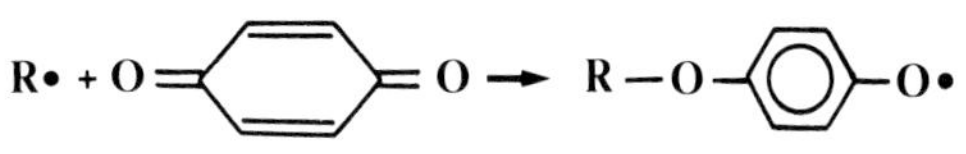

(X)   (y)   (z)

Fig. 13.2 The inhibitor (hydroquinone) (y), works by reacting with active radicals (x), to form stable radicals (z).

about polymerization of the methylmethacrylate.

The initiator present in the powder may consist of peroxide remaining unreacted after the production of the beads, in addition to extra peroxide added to the beads after their manufacture.

Polymethylmethacrylate is a clear, glass-like polymer and is occasionally used in this form for denture base construction. It is more normal, however, for manufacturers to incorporate pigments and opacifiers in order to produce a more 'lifelike' denture base. Sometimes, small fibres coated with pigment are used to give a veined appearance. Pink pigments used in denture base resins are traditionally salts of cadmium. These pigments have good colour stability and have been shown to leach cadmium from the denture base in only minute amounts. Fears over the toxicity of cadmium compounds, however, have led to the gradual replacement of cadmium salts with other 'safer' substances.

The major component of the liquid is methylmethacrylate (MMA) monomer. This is a clear, colourless, low-viscosity liquid with a boiling point of 100·3°C and a distinct odour exaggerated by a relatively high vapour pressure at room temperature. MMA is one of a group of monomers which are very susceptible to free radical addition polymerization (Fig. 12.3). Following mixing of the powder and liquid components and activation by either heat or chemical means, the *curing* of the denture base material is due to the polymerization of MMA monomer to form polymethylmethacrylate.

The liquid normally contains some cross-linking agent. The substance most widely used is ethyleneglycoldimethacrylate, the structural formula of which is given in Fig. 12.7. This compound is used to improve the physical properties of the set material.

The inhibitor is used to prolong the *shelf life* of the liquid component. In the absence of inhibitor, polymerization of monomer and cross-linking agent would occur slowly, even at room temperature and below, due to the random occurrence of free radicals within the liquid. The source of these free radicals is uncertain, but once formed they cause a slow increase in viscosity of the liquid and may eventually cause the liquid component to set solid.

The inhibitor, which is commonly a derivative of hydroquinone, works by reacting rapidly with radicals formed within the liquid to form stabilized radicals which are not capable of initiating polymerization. This is illustrated in Fig. 13.2 in which the product radical (z) is a relatively stable species which will not initiate polymerization of MMA at room temperature. The stability of the radical (z) is explained by the fact that the unpaired electron is not isolated in the oxygen atom but may occupy several sites around the ring, as shown in Fig. 13.3.

One way of reducing the occurrence of unwanted radicals in the liquid is to store the material in a can or in a dark-brown bottle. Visible light or ultraviolet radiation may activate compounds which are potentially capable of forming radicals. Eliminating the source of radiation is therefore beneficial.

The activator is present only in those products which are described as *self-curing* or *cold curing* materials and not in *heat curing* denture base materials. The function of the activator is to react with the peroxide in the powder to create free radicals which can initiate polymerization of the monomer.

Mixing and curing (heat curing materials)

Mixing The manipulation of acrylic denture base materials involves the mixing of powder and liquid to form a 'dough' which is 'packed' into a gypsum mould for curing. The ratio of powder to liquid is important since it controls the 'workability' of the

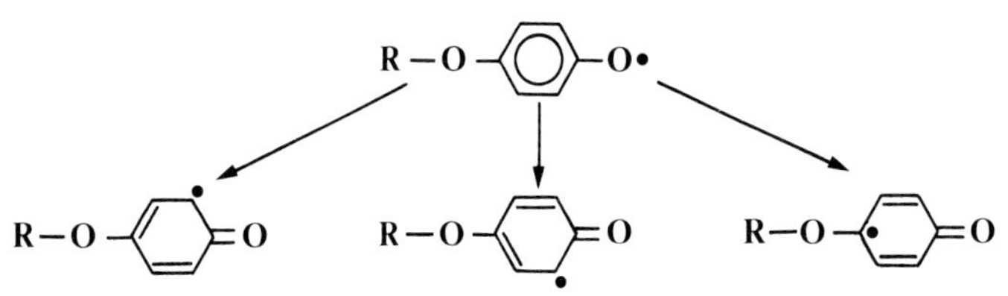

R-O-⟨◯⟩-O•

R-O-⟨⟩=O   R-O-⟨⟩=O   R-O-⟨⟩=O

Fig. 13.3 The stability of the radical (z) formed in Fig. 13.2 is explained by the way in which the unpaired electron can occupy several sites in the molecule.

mix as well as the dimensional change on setting. Methylmethacrylate monomer undergoes a volumetric polymerization shrinkage of 21 percent on conversion to polymer. This shrinkage is considerably reduced by using a mix with a high powder/liquid ratio. If the powder/liquid ratio is too high however, the mix becomes 'dry' and unmanageable and the mixture will not flow when placed under pressure in the gypsum mould. In addition, there is insufficient monomer in a dry mix to bind all the polymer beads together. This may produce a granular effect on the denture surface which is normally referred to as *granular porosity*.

In order to produce a workable mix, whilst maintaining shrinkage at a low level, a powder/liquid ratio of 2·5:1 by weight is normally used. This gives a volumetric polymerization shrinkage of around 5−6 percent.

Proportioning is normally carried out by placing a suitable volume of liquid into a clean, dry mixing vessel followed by slow addition of powder, allowing each powder particle to become *wetted* by monomer. The mixture is then stirred and left to stand until it reaches a consistency suitable for packing into the gypsum mould. During this standing period, a lid should be placed on the mixing vessel to prevent evaporation of monomer. Loss of monomer during this stage could produce *granular porosity* in the set material. This is characterized by a blotchy, opaque surface.

Immediately after mixing, a material of rather 'sandy' consistency is produced. After a short period of time this becomes a 'sticky' mass which forms 'strings' of material, sticking to the spatula, if an attempt is made to carry out further mixing. The next stage is the 'dough' stage. Here, the material is more cohesive and has lost much of its 'tackiness'. It can be moulded like plasticine and does not adhere to the sides of the mixing vessel. The material should be packed into the mould at this stage. If packing is delayed the material may become quite tough and rubbery and eventually becomes quite hard.

The transitions from 'sandy' to 'stringy' to 'dough' and eventually rubbery and hard stages are

due to physical changes occurring within the mix. Smaller polymer beads dissolve in monomer causing a gradual increase in viscosity of the liquid phase. Larger beads absorb monomer and swell, thus depriving the liquid phase of monomer and causing a further increase in viscosity. During this period the monomer remains unpolymerized.

The time taken to reach the dough stage is called the *doughing time* whilst the time for which the material remains at the dough stage and is mouldable is termed the *working time*. Manufacturers aim to combine a short doughing time with a long working time. They do this by controlling such factors as bead size and molecular weight of the powder. Smaller beads, with lower molecular weight, dissolve more rapidly in the polymer.

The dough is packed into a two-part gypsum mould, which has previously been treated with a mould-sealing compound (Fig. 13.4). Excess dough is used and a *trial closure* is performed causing excess material to form a 'flash' at the point where the two halves of the flask meet. The flask is opened and the 'flash' removed. The flask is then closed again under pressure using a threaded bench press and maintained under pressure during curing using a spring-loaded clamp. The applied pressure has three important functions. It ensures that

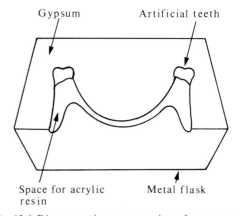

Fig. 13.4 Diagrammatic representation of two-part split mould used for acrylic denture construction.

'dough' flows into every part of the mould. It enables excess 'dough' to be used thus causing an effective reduction in the polymerization shrinkage and it prevents the formation of a 'raised bite' on the denture by giving a base which is too thick.

The use of insufficient dough to create an excess in the mould or the application of insufficient pressure during curing can lead to porosity voids dispersed throughout the whole mass of the denture base. This is known as *contraction porosity*.

Occasionally, the dough is forced into the mould by *injection moulding*. A sprue hole and a vent hole are formed in the gypsum mould and the metal flask is constructed such that it will adapt to the injection moulding equipment. During processing, the equipment is normally arranged so that a 'wave' of curing propagates from the part of the flask which is furthest from the sprue and vents. This enables shrinkage during curing to be compensated by taking up extra material from the sprue reservoir.

Curing Having filled the mould with dough, the next stage is to polymerize the monomer to produce the final 'processed' denture. Curing is normally carried out by placing the clamped flask in either a water bath or an air oven. Whichever type of system is used, many 'curing cycles' are available. When choosing which curing cycle to use, attention should be paid to certain facts:

(1) Benzoyl peroxide initiator begins to decompose rapidly to form free radicals above 65°C,

(2) The polymerization reaction is highly exothermic,

(3) The boiling point of the monomer is 100·3°C and if the temperature of the dough is raised significantly above this, the monomer will boil, producing spherical voids in the hottest part of the curing dough. These will be apparent as *gaseous porosity* in the cured denture base (Fig. 13.5),

(4) It is important to get a high degree of conversion from monomer to polymer and to produce a polymer with high molecular weight. Residual monomer and low molecular weight polymer result in poor mechanical properties as well as possible adverse tissue reactions.

Taking the above points into account, manufacturers often recommend curing cycles which they feel are appropriate for their brand of denture base material.

One popular method is to heat the flask containing the dough for seven hours at 70°C followed by three hours at 100°C. Most of the conversion of monomer to polymer occurs during the 7 hours at 70°C stage, during which time the temperature of the dough itself may approach 100°C due to the polymerization exotherm (Fig. 13.6a). The final 3 hours at 100°C ensure almost complete conversion of monomer in those thinner areas of the denture base where the effect of the exothermic heat of reaction is less pronounced. There are many other curing cycles which manufacturers recommend and it is not possible to list all of them. One other example is to place the flask in a bath of cold water. The water is gradually brought to the boil over a period of one hour, allowed to boil for one hour and then allowed to cool slowly. Very few manufacturers recommend that the flask, containing dough, is placed directly into boiling water since this, coupled with the exothermic heat of reaction, can cause the dough to reach temperatures, in excess of 150°C as shown in Fig. 13.6b. This would, undoubtedly, result in *gaseous porosity* being produced in the thicker parts of the denture.

Before deflasking the processed denture the flask is cooled to room temperature. This may lead to the setting up of internal stresses within the denture base since the coefficient of thermal expansion of acrylic resin is about 10 times greater than that of the gypsum mould material. These internal stresses may be compounded with those caused by polymerization shrinkage, although the latter are normally eliminated by plastic flow when the polymerization takes place at elevated temperatures. Internal stresses may lead to warpage of the denture base at a later stage if the denture is placed in warm water for cleaning. The magnitude of the stresses can be reduced by allowing the flask to cool slowly from the curing temperature.

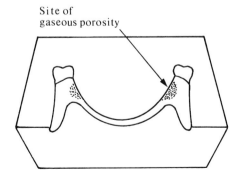

Site of
gaseous porosity

Fig. 13.5 Diagram illustrating the normal sites of gaseous porosity in an upper denture.

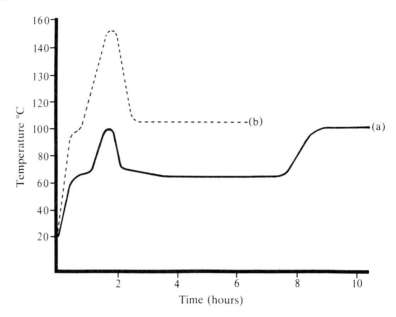

Fig. 13.6 Curing cycles (temperature versus time) for heat curing acrylic denture resins. (a) The curing flask is placed in an oven or water bath at 70°C for 7 hours. The temperature is raised to 100°C for 1 hour. (b) The curing flask is placed directly into an oven or water bath at 100°C. Temperature of the acrylic dough is indicated.

Mixing and curing (cold curing materials)

When constructing a denture base from a cold curing material, powder and liquid components are mixed together just as for the heat curing products. Mixing is followed by a gradual increase in viscosity until the 'dough' stage is reached. This increase in viscosity is due to a combination of physical and chemical changes occurring in the mix. Smaller acrylic beads are dissolved in the monomer, whilst the larger beads absorb monomer and become 'swollen'. In addition, when peroxide from the powder and chemical activator from the liquid meet during mixing the polymerization of monomer is initiated. Thus, conversion of monomer to polymer contributes to the increase in viscosity. Generally, these materials reach the 'dough' stage quite quickly and remain workable for only a short period of time. Within a few minutes of attaining a 'dough' consistency, the rate of polymerization increases rapidly causing a large temperature rise and the material becomes hard and unmanageable. The time available for carrying out a trial closure of the processing flask is minimal and, if the viscosity has increased beyond a certain point at the time of final closure, there is a danger of increased vertical height in the denture. These problems, coupled with the inferior mechanical properties and higher residual monomer content of the cold curing resins,

generally restrict their use to *repairing and relining* of dentures. For repairing, a very fluid mix of cold cure resin is used. The large excess of monomer ensures adequate 'wetting' of the fragments being repaired.

Some cold cure resins, known as *pourable resins*, are occasionally used for denture base construction. These materials are mixed to a very fluid consistency using a low powder/liquid ratio. The mixed material is poured into a hydrocolloid mould and allowed to cure at or just above room temperature. The advantage of this technique is that the cured denture can be removed from the flexible hydrocolloid mould with a minimum of time and effort and the denture base needs little further finishing. The disadvantages are high residual monomer levels coupled with inferior mechanical properties of the base and the possibility of distortions arising from the use of a flexible mould.

Properties

Physical properties   From the point of view of appearance the acrylic denture base materials are adequate. The materials are available in a variety of shades and opacities and can be veined or un-veined. Characterization 'kits' containing various pigments allow tissue colour matching for patients of various races.

The value of Tg may vary from one product to another depending on the average molecular weight and the level of residual monomer. A typical value of Tg for a heat curing material is 105°C. This is somewhat higher than any temperature which the base should reach during 'normal' service. The value of modulus of elasticity decreases and the potential for creep increases considerably at temperatures approaching Tg however, and patients may cause distortions by soaking dentures in boiling water. Tg values for cold curing resins are generally lower than those for heat curing products. A value of about 90°C would be typical. Thus, there is a greater chance of these products suffering distortions in hot water. The use of water at temperatures above around 65°C should be avoided for soaking dentures. This not only ensures that the Tg of the resin is not approached but also that the relief of internal stresses, accompanied by distortions, is minimized.

Acrylic resins have relatively low values of specific gravity (approximately $1\cdot2$ g/cm^3) because they are composed of groups of 'light' atoms, for example, carbon, oxygen and hydrogen. The 'lightness' of the resulting denture is beneficial, since the gravitational forces causing displacement of an upper denture are minimized. Dentures constructed from acrylic resin are radiolucent because C, O and H atoms are poor X-ray absorbers. This is a serious disadvantage of these materials. If a patient swallows or inhales a denture or fragment of a denture it is difficult to detect using simple radiological techniques.

Acrylic resin may be considered a good thermal insulator. Its thermal conductivity is some 100–1000 times less than the values for metals and alloys. This is a disadvantage for a denture base because the oral soft tissues are denied normal thermal stimuli which help to maintain the mucosa in a healthy condition. In addition, the patient may

partially lose the protective reflex responses to hot and cold stimulii. This may result in some painful experiences, for example, when taking hot drinks.

Mechanical properties Compared with alloys such as Co/Cr and stainless steel, acrylic resins would be classified as soft, weak and flexible materials (Table 13.2). Providing the denture base is constructed in sufficient thickness however, rigidity and strength are adequate. Dentures are subjected to bending forces and the flexural stress required to cause fracture depends on the square of the thickness of the denture (p. 7). Thus, if the thickness of the base is doubled, the stress required to fracture is increased fourfold. Although this factor is important it can be applied to only a limited extent when designing an acrylic denture base since a thick base may be more difficult for the patient to tolerate and will further increase the degree of thermal insulation. The transverse strength of acrylic is generally sufficient to resist fracture caused by the application of a high masticatory load. Fractures of dentures, *in situ*, do occur however, as a result of fatigue. This is often the result of a patient wearing an ill-fitting or badly designed denture which flexes considerably with each masticatory load. Acrylic resin has a relatively poor resistance to fatigue fracture, a fact which is mainly responsible for the large number of denture repairs which are carried out annually.

Acrylic resin also has a relatively poor impact strength and if a denture is dropped onto a hard surface there is a high probability of fracture occurring.

Crazing may sometimes appear on the surface of an acrylic denture. This is a series of surface cracks which may have a weakening effect on the base. The cracks may arise by one of three mechanisms. If the patient develops the habit of frequently removing his denture and allowing it to dry out, the constant cycle of water absorption followed by drying may develop sufficient tensile stresses at the

Table 13.2 Mechanical properties of acrylic resin (a comparison with certain alloys)

	Modulus of elasticity* GPa	Tensile strength* MPa	Hardness* VHN
Acrylic resin	$2\cdot5$	85	20
Co/Cr	220	850	420
Stainless steel	220	1000	400

*Values given are typical values. There may be significant variations between products.

surface to cause crazing. Thus, patients are instructed to keep their dentures moist at all times. The use of porcelain teeth may cause crazing of the base in the region around the tooth neck due to differences in the coefficient of thermal expansion between porcelain and acrylic resin (ratio about 1:10). Thirdly, crazing may arise during denture repair when methylmethacrylate monomer contacts the cured acrylic resin of the fragments being repaired. One function of the cross-linking agent is to reduce the degree of crazing by binding polymer chains together.

Vickers hardness numbers (Table 13.2) indicate that acrylic polymers are relatively soft, especially when compared to alloys. This predisposes the acrylic denture base to wear, caused by abrasive foodstuffs and particularly abrasive dentifrice cleansers. Wear of the denture base arises as a serious problem on very few occasions however and cannot be considered as a major disadvantage of acrylic resin denture materials. Dentifrices can be graded in terms of abrasivity depending on the type and particle size of the abrasive used. Whilst it would seem prudent to select a dentifrice of low abrasivity for cleaning dentures, it should be realized that some abrasive power is probably required in order to achieve adequate cleaning.

Chemical and biological properties Acrylic resin slowly absorbs water and an equilibrium value of about 2 percent absorption is reached after a period of several days or weeks depending on the thickness of the denture. Loss or gain of water in the surface layers may occur quite rapidly however — a fact which contributes towards surface crazing.

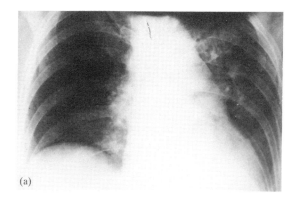

(a)

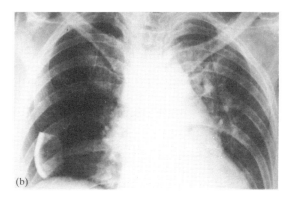

(b)

Fig. 13.7 Chest radiographs in which a segment of denture base has been placed over the lower right half of the chest: (a) for a radiolucent denture base material; (b) for a radiopaque denture base material. (From *Journal of Dentistry* (1976) vol. **4**, p. 214 with permission.)

Absorption of water causes a dimensional change, although this may be considered insignificant. This has never been demonstrated as a major cause of ill-fitting dentures in the presently available materials.

Associated with water absorption is the ability of certain organisms to colonize the fitting surface of an acrylic denture. It is not clear whether organisms, such as *Candida albicans*, exist entirely *on* the surface of the denture or whether they penetrate the outer layers of resin. Frequent cleansing, coupled with the practice of soaking dentures overnight, is normally sufficient to prevent the growth of these unwanted organisms and their associated clinical problems, such as *denture stomatitis*.

A very small minority of patients are reported to be *allergic* to acrylic resin and in particular to the

Table 13.3 Radiopaque denture base materials

Radiopaque additive	Comments
Metal inserts or powdered metals	May weaken base and appearance is poor.
Inorganic salts such as barium sulphate	Insufficient radiopacity at low concentrations. Weaken base at high concentrations.
Comonomers containing heavy metals e.g. barium acrylate	Polymer has poor mechanical properties.
Halogen-containing comonomers or additives e.g. tribromophenyl-methacrylate	Additives may act as plasticizers. Comonomers are expensive.

residual methylmethacrylate monomer which may exist within the base. When such cases can be proved genuine, it is necessary to use an alternative material. Patients who are not allergic may, nevertheless, suffer *irritation* if very high levels of monomer exist in, say, an undercured denture base.

Acrylic resin should be treated with respect and handled with care by technicians involved in its manipulation. Levels of acrylic powder dust and methylmethacrylate monomer in the atmosphere should both be kept to a minimum since both may be potentially harmful.

13.4 Modified acrylic materials

The majority of acrylic resin is used in the unmodified form as discussed in Section 13.3. Some products have been developed, however, in which attempts have been made to improve impact strength, fatigue resistance or radiopacity.

The impact strength of acrylic polymers can be significantly improved by the incorporation of elastomers. The elastomer is able to absorb energy on impact and thus protect the acrylic resin from fracture. An alternative to the direct addition of elastomers is the use of acrylic–elastomer copolymers. These are, typically, methylmethacrylate–butadiene or methylmethacrylate–butadiene-styrene copolymers which are now available in certain commercial products. Despite the fact that impact strength can be increased almost tenfold in this way, these polymers are not widely used, mainly because of their greater cost.

One attempt to improve the fatigue resistance of acrylic denture polymers has involved the use of carbon fibre inserts. If the fibres are correctly positioned they may have a beneficial effect. They stiffen the denture, reducing the degree of flexing and the possibility of fatigue fracture. They also considerably increase the flexural strength. The technique is not in widespread use however, for several reasons. In order to gain benefit from the fibres, the positioning is critical. They must be placed in that part of the denture which is under a tensile stress. Bonding between the fibres and the acrylic resin may be difficult to achieve and if bonding is not achieved the fibres may 'weaken' the denture. The technique adds a complicating factor to the

denture construction process and, finally, the appearance of the denture is adversely affected because the carbon fibres are black.

There have been many attempts to incorporate a degree of radiopacity into acrylic denture base materials. Table 13.3 summarizes the methods which have been suggested. Each method involves the incorporation of atoms of higher atomic number than the C, H and O atoms of which acrylic resin is comprised. One commercially available product contained 8 percent barium sulphate. This did not produce sufficient levels of radiopacity. Increasing the barium sulphate content to a level of 20 percent gives sufficient radiopacity but unfortunately has a deleterious effect on the mechanical properties of the resin. The most promising materials under development appear to be those in which bromine-containing additives or comonomers are used to give radiopacity. Fig. 13.7 shows chest radiographs in which a segment of a denture has been placed over the lower right chest area. In the case of a conventional denture base material the denture segment is not visible on the radiograph. A material with a bromine-containing additive is clearly visible.

13.5 Alternative polymers

The major alternatives to acrylic polymers or modified acrylics are the polycarbonates and certain vinyl polymers. These may be considered when the patient has a proven allergy to acrylic resin or when greater impact strength is required. The polycarbonates and some of the vinyl polymers are processed by injection moulding and so can only be used when the specialist equipment is available.

Polycarbonates have Tg values around 150°C and are generally moulded at temperatures well in excess of this. Consequently, the moulded base may have internal stresses after moulding and is likely to distort if placed in hot water. Some of the vinyl resins, on the other hand, have very low softening temperatures, as low as 60°C in some cases. These must obviously be handled with care if distortions are to be avoided.

The other alternative to acrylic resin is vulcanite. The equipment required for processing a vulcanite denture is now a rarity, however, and the material can no longer be considered as a serious alternative.

14   Denture Lining Materials

14.1 Introduction

Denture lining materials are of several types and are used for a variety of reasons. Occasionally, the fitting surface of an acrylic denture needs replacement in order to improve the fit of the denture. In this case, there are two options. Either the whole of the denture base can be replaced with fresh heat curing acrylic resin, or a lining of a self-curing resin may be applied to the fitting surface of the existing base.

Sometimes it is necessary to apply a very soft material to the fitting surface of a denture in order to act as a 'cushion' which will enable traumatized soft tissues to recover before recording an impression for a new denture.

Some patients are unable to tolerate a 'hard' denture base and must be provided with a 'permanent' soft cushion on the fitting surface of the denture.

Table 14.1 Composition of typical hard reline materials

Type 1	*Powder*	
	Polymer beads	Polymethylmeth-acrylate
	Initiator	Benzoyl peroxide
	Pigments	Probably inorganic salt
	Liquid	
	Monomer	Methylmethacrylate
	Plasticizer	Di-*n*-butylphthalate
	Chemical activator	Tertiary amine
Type 2	*Powder*	
	Polymer beads	Polyethylmethacrylate
	Initiator	Benzoyl peroxide
	Pigments	Probably inorganic salt
	Liquid	
	Monomer	Butylmethacrylate
	Chemical activator	Tertiary amine

The materials which satisfy the various requirements listed above can be classified into three groups as follows:

(1) Hard reline materials,
(2) Tissue conditioners,
(3) Soft lining materials.

14.2 Hard reline materials

The materials discussed in this section are those products which are used to provide a 'chairside' reline to the denture. The method should be distinguished from laboratory relining and *rebasing* techniques which involve replacing most of the denture base resin with fresh, heat cured polymer.

Composition The materials are generally supplied as a powder and liquid which are mixed together. Table 14.1 gives the composition of the two types of material in common use. The major difference between the two types is that the liquid in the type 1 material contains methylmethacrylate monomer, whilst the liquid of the type 2 material contains butylmethacrylate monomer. Both type 1 and type 2 materials may be classified as 'cold curing' resins and will readily polymerize at room temperature or mouth temperature.

Manipulation The normal procedure is to 'relieve' the fitting surface of the denture by grinding away some of the hard acrylic denture base. The powder and liquid of the hard reline material are then mixed in the recommended proportions to give a fluid mix of material. This is applied to the fitting surface of the denture which is seated in the patient's mouth whilst still fluid. The impression is then recorded with the dentures in occlusion. The reline material soon becomes rubbery and the impression of the patient's soft tissues is recorded.

The denture is then removed from the patient's mouth and allowed to bench cure. Setting may be accelerated by placing the denture in warm water. The materials are not allowed to remain in the patient's mouth throughout setting since the exothermic heat of reaction may cause an unbearably high temperature rise. The relined denture is normally ready for trimming and polishing within 30 minutes.

Properties The major disadvantage of the type 1 materials is that they involve direct contact between the oral soft tissues and a fluid mixture of reline material containing methylmethacrylate monomer. The latter material is known to be irritant and may also sensitize patients who may then suffer allergic responses in the future. The advice offered by some manufacturers, to smear the soft tissues with petroleum jelly prior to recording the impression, is probably inadequate.

The type 2 materials contain butylmethacrylate monomer in the liquid component. This is known to be a far less irritant substance than methylmethacrylate.

Both type 1 and type 2 materials have low values of glass transition temperature (Tg). The reasons for this are the presence of plasticizer in type 1 materials and the use of higher methacrylates (ethyl and butyl) in the type 2 materials. This may lead to increased dimensional instability in the relined denture, particularly if the existing hard base has been significantly relieved in order to accommodate the lining.

The reline materials are often porous due to air inclusions during mixing of the powder and liquid. The initial fluidity of the mix, coupled with a relatively rapid increase in viscosity during setting at atmospheric pressure, ensure that it is difficult to eliminate voids. This is often considered unsightly and may affect patient acceptance.

One criticism of the direct reline materials is that the dentist has little control over the thickness of the lining achieved and therefore over the 'height' of the denture. This is an important point since increasing the thickness of the denture base may reduce the freeway space.

It follows that the direct reline materials should be considered as only a temporary or at best semipermanent solution to the problem of an ill-fitting denture.

14.3 Tissue conditioners

Tissue conditioners are soft denture liners which may be applied to the fitting surface of a denture. They are used to provide a temporary cushion which prevents masticatory loads from being transferred to the underlying hard and soft tissues.

Tissue conditioners have several applications. For example, when the soft tissues have become traumatized due to wearing an ill-fitting denture the dentist would like the tissues to recover before recording impressions for new dentures. Ideally, the patient would refrain from wearing his denture for a period, but this is not popular. In these circumstances, a layer of a cushioning tissue conditioner on the fitting surface of the denture will enable the soft tissues to recover without depriving the patient of his dignity.

Tissue conditioners are often applied to the dentures of patients who have undergone surgery. This reduces pain and helps prevent traumatization of the wound.

Another application of tissue conditioners is as *functional impression materials*. A layer of tissue conditioner in the fitting surface of the denture enables a functional impression to be obtained over a period of a few days.

Requirements Tissue conditioners should remain *soft* during use in order to maintain an adequate cushioning effect on the underlying soft tissues. The material should be *resilient* in order that masticatory loads are absorbed without causing permanent deformation of the lining. Paradoxically, when the materials are being used to obtain a functional impression a degree of *permanent deformation* under load is required. This enables the impression of the soft tissues to be altered during normal function.

Composition The materials are normally supplied as powder and liquid components which are mixed together. Table 14.2 gives the composition of a typical product. The relative amounts of solvent and plasticizer in the liquid component vary from one product to another. The powder is generally unpigmented, giving a white lining which is easily distinguishable from the pink denture base.

It is important to note that the liquid component contains no monomer and the powder no initiator. When the powder and liquid are mixed together, a

Table 14.2 Composition of a tissue conditioner

Powder		
	Polymer beads	Polyethylmethacrylate
Liquid		
	Solvent	Ethyl alcohol
	Plasticizer	Butylphthalyl butylglycolate

purely physical process occurs. The solvent dissolves the smaller polymer beads and the larger beads become swollen with solvent which acts as a carrier for the plasticizer. The final 'set' material is gel-like, with swollen, plasticized spheres being cemented together with a matrix which is a saturated solution of polymer in a solvent/plasticizer mixture. The 'softness' of the set material is a function of the use of a higher methacrylate, ethylmethacrylate, coupled with considerable quantities of plasticizer and solvent.

Manipulation Tissue conditioners are used in chairside techniques in which the freshly mixed material is applied to the fitting surface of the denture. The denture is then seated in the patient's mouth, whilst the conditioner is still in a fluid state, in order to obtain an impression of the soft tissues. This stage of the procedure is important, since the aim is to form a cushion of reasonable thickness so that it will be effective, but not to increase the 'height' of the denture unduly compared to the unlined denture. On completion of setting the tissue conditioner should ideally form a regular layer over the whole of the fitting surface of the denture. It is normal practice to inspect the denture and the patient's soft tissues after 2−3 days to ascertain whether the tissue conditioning has been successful or, alternatively, whether an adequate functional impression has been obtained.

Properties Tissue conditioners are initially very soft, having a modulus of elasticity value around 0·05 MPa after one hour compared with a value of 2000 MPa for normal acrylic denture base materials. They do not remain permanently soft however, since the alcohol and plasticizer are leached rapidly into saliva. The time taken for the materials to become so hard that they no longer give adequate cushioning varies from a few days to a week or two, depending upon the product used. Those materials which are softer initially, harden more rapidly and

vice versa. For adequate conditioning, with a very soft material, the conditioner should be replaced with fresh material every 2−3 days until the tissues have recovered.

The materials are able to perform the functions of both a tissue conditioner and functional impression material due to their *viscoelastic* properties. The apparent paradox of requiring an elastic material for one purpose and a plastic one for the other is overcome in this way. The viscoelastic properties of the materials may be described by the Maxwell and Voigt models in series as discussed on p. 14 and illustrated in Fig. 2.15. The elastic nature of the products is extremely time-dependent. Under the influence of dynamic forces which are applied for a second or less during mastication, the materials are essentially elastic and provide a cushioning effect. Each application of force does, however, cause a small permanent deformation which helps to record the functional impression. Under the influence of smaller, resting loads, further permanent deformation occurs.

One of the most important properties of these materials is that they are non-irritant due to the absence of acrylic monomers from the liquid component.

14.4 Temporary soft lining materials
These materials are very similar to the tissue conditioners. They are supplied as a powder and liquid, the composition of which is equivalent to that given in Table 14.2. The materials are not as soft as the tissue conditioners immediately after setting but they retain their softness for longer, taking up to a month or two to harden. Like the tissue conditioners, they are viscoelastic in nature and give a cushioning effect under dynamic conditions of loading.

The method of manipulation of these products is similar to that discussed for tissue conditioners, but because they take longer to harden they do not require replacing as frequently. Care should be exercised when selecting a denture cleanser to use with a denture carrying a temporary soft lining or tissue conditioner. The oxygenating-type cleansers, in particular, cause surface degradation and pitting of the materials.

Temporary soft liners are often used in place of tissue conditioners in cases where it is not practicable to replace the conditioner every 2−3 days. In

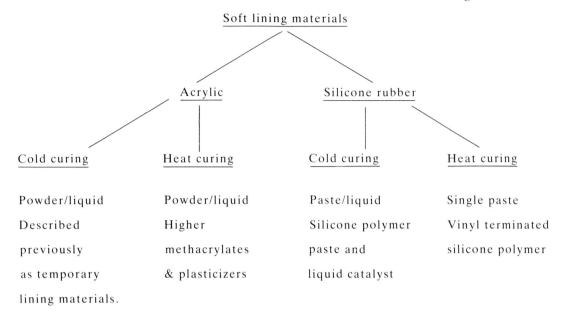

Fig. 14.1 Soft lining materials. An indication of the type of materials which are available.

addition, they may be used as a means of temporarily improving the fit of an ill-fitting denture until such a time as a new denture can be constructed. Another use of the products is as a diagnostic aid to ascertain whether the patient would benefit from a permanent soft lining.

14.5 Permanent soft lining materials

Permanent soft lining materials are most commonly used for patients who cannot tolerate a hard base. This problem generally arises if the patient has an irregular mandibular ridge covered by a thin and relatively non-resilient mucosa. Not surprisingly it may be very painful when a masticatory load is applied through a hard base on to this type of supporting tissue. In such cases, a soft lining on the denture will help to relieve the pain and increase patient acceptance of the denture.

Requirements The requirements of a permanent soft lining are more critical than those of the tissue conditioner and temporary lining materials since they are expected to function over a much longer period of time.

The materials used should be permanently soft, ideally for the lifetime of the denture. They should be elastic in order to give a cushioning effect and prevent unacceptable distortions during service. The lining should adhere to the denture base. The materials should be non-toxic, non-irritant and incapable of sustaining the growth of harmful bacteria or fungi.

Available materials Fig. 14.1 indicates the types of materials which are available for use as permanent soft linings. Those products described as cold curing acrylic materials are in fact the materials which are described as temporary soft lining materials. These materials harden within a period of a few weeks or at best a few months and cannot therefore be seriously considered as permanent soft linings since they would require regular replacement. One advantage of these materials is that they can be readily applied to an existing denture, by the dentist, in a chairside technique.

The heat curing acrylic materials are processed in the laboratory and are normally applied to a new denture at the time of production. They are supplied as a powder and liquid, the composition of which vary from one product to another. They rely,

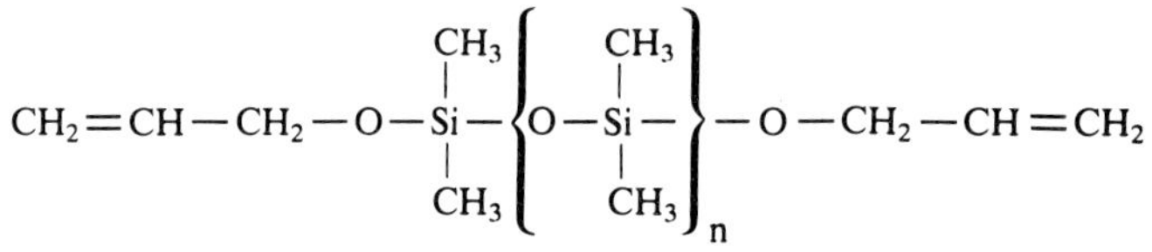

$$CH_2=CH-CH_2-O-\underset{\underset{CH_3}{|}}{\overset{\overset{CH_3}{|}}{Si}}-\left\{O-\underset{\underset{CH_3}{|}}{\overset{\overset{CH_3}{|}}{Si}}-\right\}_n-O-CH_2-CH=CH_2$$

(a) Silicone polymer with terminal vinyl groups

$$CH_2=CH-CH_2-M-CH_2-CH=CH_2$$

(b) Simplified structure of silicone polymer

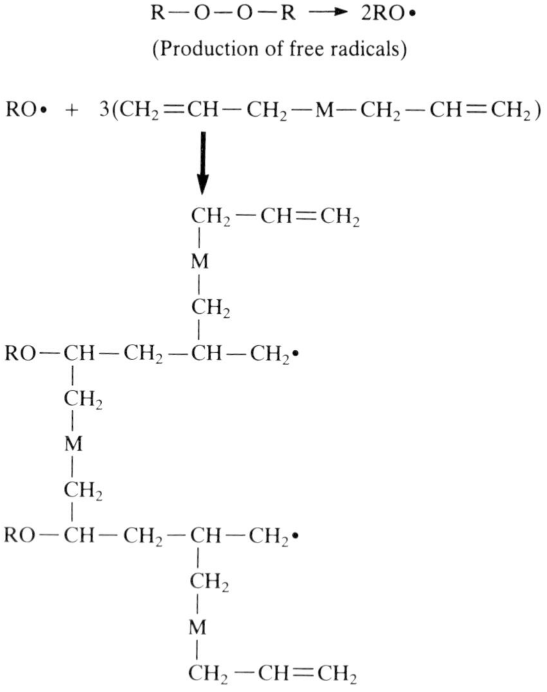

$$R-O-O-R \longrightarrow 2RO\bullet$$

(Production of free radicals)

$$RO\bullet \ + \ 3(CH_2=CH-CH_2-M-CH_2-CH=CH_2)$$

$$\downarrow$$

$$\begin{array}{l} CH_2-CH=CH_2 \\ | \\ M \\ | \\ CH_2 \\ | \\ RO-CH-CH_2-CH-CH_2\bullet \\ \quad\quad | \\ \quad\quad CH_2 \\ \quad\quad | \\ \quad\quad M \\ \quad\quad | \\ \quad\quad CH_2 \\ \quad\quad | \\ RO-CH-CH_2-CH-CH_2\bullet \\ \quad\quad\quad | \\ \quad\quad\quad CH_2 \\ \quad\quad\quad | \\ \quad\quad\quad M \\ \quad\quad\quad | \\ \quad\quad\quad CH_2-CH=CH_2 \end{array}$$

(c) First stages of the cross-linking reaction

Fig. 14.2 Vinyl-terminated (heat curing) silicone soft lining materials. (a) Vinyl-terminated silicone prepolymer (mixed with inert filler to form paste). (b) Simplified formula of prepolymer. (c) Cross-linking by a free radical mechanism, initiated by peroxide. The peroxide is activated by heating.

for softness, on the combined use of a higher methacrylate and a plasticizer. A typical powder consists of beads of polyethyl- or polybutylmethacrylate along with some peroxide initiator and pigment. The liquid is likely to be a mixture of butylmethacrylate and plasticizer. Powder and liquid are mixed to form a type of 'dough' which is heat processed simultaneously with the hard acrylic base.

A similar technique is used when applying a heat curing silicone soft lining. These products are supplied as a single paste which consists of a polydimethylsiloxane polymer with pendant or terminal vinyl groups through which cross-linking takes place. The liquid polymer is formulated into a paste by adding inert fillers such as silica. The paste

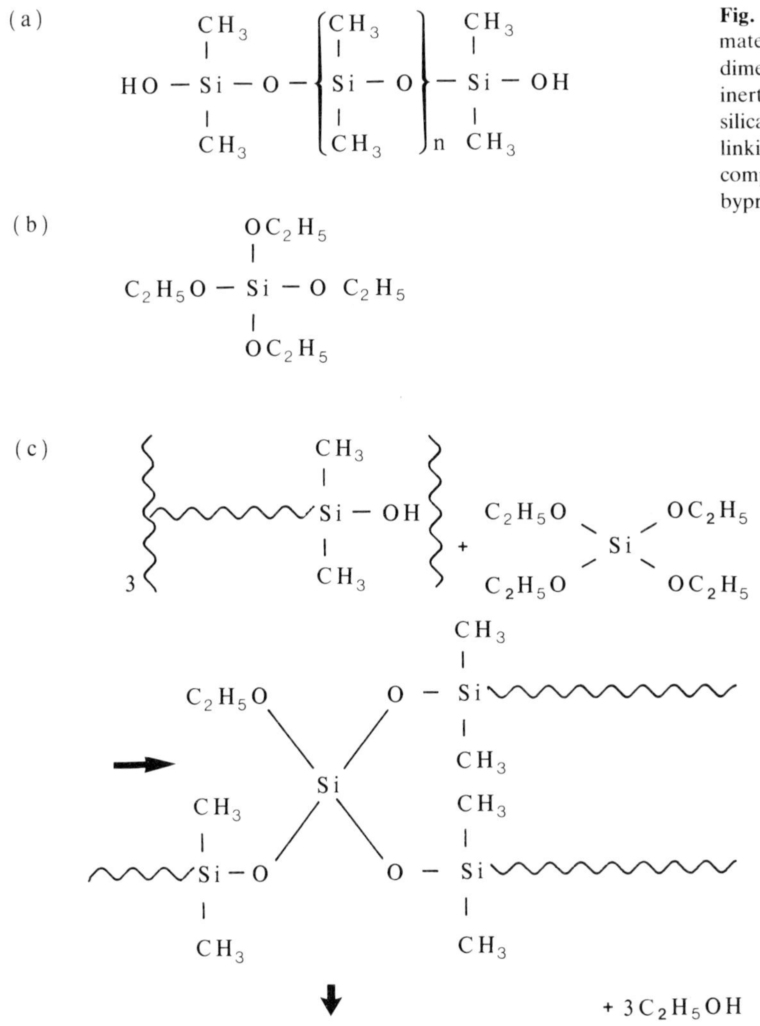

(a)

(b)

(c)

Fig. 14.3 Cold curing silicone soft lining materials. (a) Hydroxyl-terminated polydimethylsiloxane prepolymer (mixed with inert filler to form paste). (b) Tetraethylsilicate (cross-linking agent). (c) Cross-linking reaction, catalysed by a tin compound. Ethyl alcohol is liberated as a byproduct.

also contains a free radical initiator such as a peroxide which breaks down on heating to initiate the cross-linking reaction. Fig. 14.2 illustrates the structural formula and mechanism of cross-linking of the vinyl-terminated silicone polymer.

The cold curing silicone products are supplied as a paste and liquid. The paste contains a hydroxyl-terminated polydimethylsiloxane liquid polymer (Fig. 14.3a) and inert filler. The liquid contains a mixture of a cross-linking agent, such as tetraethyl silicate (Fig. 14.3b) and a catalyst which is normally an organo-tin compound such as dibutyl tin dilaurate. On mixing the paste and liquid a condensation cross-linking reaction takes place. Alcohol is produced as a byproduct of this reaction

(Fig. 14.3c). Cross-linking causes the paste to be converted to a rubber.

Although the cold curing silicones are cured at room temperature, they are generally processed in the laboratory. The method normally used is to pour casts into the dentures. The casts with dentures are then mounted on an articulator and the fitting surface of the dentures is relieved to make space for the lining. The paste and liquid are mixed together and the fluid mix applied to the fitting surface of the dentures. The dentures are then repositioned on the casts, the articulator closed into occlusion and the material allowed to set. An alternative method is to use an overcast instead of an articulator.

Properties   All four types of soft lining material are sufficiently soft on insertion to give an adequate cushioning effect. The softest of the four materials initially are the cold curing acrylic materials. These products harden, however, through rapid loss of alcohol and slow leaching of plasticizer. The heat curing acrylic products, though not as soft as the cold curing products initially, retain their softness for longer. They too eventually become hard due to gradual leaching of plasticizer into the oral fluids. The silicone materials remain permanently soft and the modulus of elasticity value may, in fact, decrease due to water absorption. This may cause problems with some silicones since water absorption may be followed by bacterial or fungal growth in the soft lining. The silicones have good elastic properties and retain their shape after setting despite being subjected to masticatory loading. The acrylic materials, on the other hand, are visco-elastic and gradually become distorted. There is a tendency for the materials to 'flow away' from areas of greatest stress causing the cushioning effect to be lost.

The durability of the bond between the denture base and the soft lining is adequate for the acrylic materials and the heat cured silicone products. In the case of the cold curing silicone material, however, there is a tendency for the lining to peel away from the base. This occurs despite the use of an adhesion primer supplied by the manufacturers. The problem is often reduced by 'boxing in' the soft lining.

Some soft linings are adversely affected by denture cleansers. Oxygenating cleansers may cause surface pitting in acrylic linings whilst brushing accelerates the rate at which silicone soft linings become detached. Soaking in a very *dilute* solution of hypochlorite is probably the most acceptable way of achieving denture hygiene without damaging the soft lining.

None of the soft lining materials can be considered truly permanent in nature since none could be expected to last the full lifetime of a denture. Therefore, regular reviews of patients with soft linings are essential.

15   Artificial Teeth

15.1 Introduction

Chaps. 13 and 14 have dealt with materials which are used to form the denture base and to line the fitting surface of the denture base. The other main components of a denture are the artificial teeth themselves. The materials most widely used for manufacturing artificial teeth are acrylic resin and porcelain.

15.2 Requirements

The most important requirement of artificial teeth is good appearance. They should, ideally, be indistinguishable from natural teeth in shape, colour and translucency. Good matching often requires that the shade and translucency of the artificial tooth should vary from the tip of the crown to the gingival area.

There should be good attachment between the artificial teeth and the denture base. The introduction of artificial teeth into the base should not adversely affect the base material. That is, the artificial tooth and base materials should be compatible.

It is an advantage for the artificial teeth to be of low density in order that they do not increase the weight of the denture unduly. The artificial teeth should be strong and tough in order to resist fracture. They should be hard enough to resist abrasive forces in the mouth and during cleaning, but should allow grinding with a dental bur so that adjustments to the occlusion can be made by the dentist at the chairside.

15.3 Available materials

The two materials which are commonly used for the production of artificial teeth are acrylic resins and porcelain.

Acrylic resins

Acrylic resin artificial teeth are produced in re-usable metal moulds using either the *dough moulding* technique, described for denture base construction (Chap. 13), or by *injection moulding* in which the acrylic powder is softened by heating and forced into the mould under pressure.

The resins used are highly cross-linked in order to produce artificial teeth which are resistant to crazing. The main difference between the materials and those used for denture base construction is the incorporation of tooth-coloured pigments rather than pink ones.

Porcelain

The composition and manipulation of porcelain are dealt with in Chap. 11. Artificial porcelain teeth are produced to standard shapes and sizes by using moulds which are approximately 30 percent larger than required, in order to allow for shrinkage during firing. Small holes or metal pins are incorporated in the base of the porcelain teeth during their production. These are used to give mechanical attachment to the denture base.

15.4 Properties

Both acrylic and porcelain teeth can be made to give a realistic appearance. The slightly greater translucency and depth of colour achieved with porcelain possibly gives this material a slight advantage in terms of aesthetics. Both materials are produced to a variety of shapes, sizes, colours and shades which enable selection of teeth to suit most individuals.

One aspect of porcelain teeth which is sometimes unpopular with patients is the 'clicking' sound which is made when two porcelain teeth come into contact.

Table 15.1 Some properties of artificial teeth

	Acrylic resin	Porcelain
Density (g/cm^3)	1·2	2·4
Coefficient of thermal expansion (p.p.m.°C^{-1})	80	7
Modulus of elasticity (GPa)	2·5	80
Hardness (VHN)	20	500

Attachment of the teeth to the base is through a chemical union in the case of acrylic teeth and by mechanical retention for porcelain teeth. For both materials, adequate bonding is achieved only if all traces of wax from the trial denture are removed from the teeth during the 'boiling out' stage.

Chemical bonding of the acrylic teeth depends on the softening of the resin at the base of the teeth with monomer from the 'dough' of denture base material. Some manufacturers encourage this process by constructing the base and core of the artificial teeth from uncross-linked or only lightly cross-linked resin which is more readily softened. The outer 'enamel' layers of the tooth are constructed from highly cross-linked resin to prevent crazing.

Table 15.1 list some of the physical and mechanical properties of artificial teeth.

Acrylic resin teeth are, naturally, more compatible with the denture base than porcelain teeth. There is a serious mismatch in coefficient of thermal expansion and modulus of elasticity between porcelain and acrylic resin. This may lead to crazing and cracking of the denture base in the region around the base of the porcelain teeth. Porcelain has a density value about twice that of acrylic resin and dentures constructed with porcelain teeth are much heavier.

Porcelain is brittle and teeth constructed from this material are more likely to chip and fracture than acrylic teeth.

There is a vast difference in hardness between acrylic resin and porcelain. Acrylic teeth are more likely to suffer abrasion than porcelain teeth, although this does not constitute a serious problem in more than a few rare cases.

When excessive wear is evident on acrylic denture teeth, special environmental factors or patient habits are often responsible. For example, working in a dusty or gritty environment may accelerate wear if particles of grit are ground between teeth of an upper and lower denture. Likewise the use of a very abrasive material, such as pumice, for cleaning dentures may result in marked abrasion.

The extreme hardness of porcelain is a disadvantage when adjustments, requiring grinding of teeth, are necessary. With acrylic teeth, such adjustments are carried out quite simply. For porcelain teeth however, the process is difficult and results in the glaze being removed from the surface of the porcelain.

It is a clinical impression that porcelain teeth transmit higher forces to the supporting soft tissues than acrylic teeth. This is a function of the greater modulus of elasticity of porcelain.

16

Impression Materials: Classification and Requirements

16.1 Introduction

Many dental appliances are constructed outside the patient's mouth on models of the hard and/or soft tissues. The accuracy of 'fit' and the functional efficiency of the appliance depends upon how well the model replicates the natural oral tissues. The accuracy of the model depends on the accuracy of the impression in which it was cast.

The impression stage is the first of many stages involved in the production of dentures, crowns, bridges, orthodontic appliances etc. It is of great importance, therefore, that inaccuracies are minimized at this stage, otherwise they will be carried through and possibly compounded later on.

Impression materials are generally transferred to the patient's mouth in an impression 'tray'. The tray is required because the materials are initially quite fluid and require support. Once positioned in the patient's mouth, the materials undergo 'setting' by either a chemical or physical process. After 'setting', the impression is removed from the patient's mouth and the model cast using dental plaster or stone.

16.2 Classification of impression materials

Many criteria may be used to classify impression materials. One simple method is to refer to materials by their generic chemical name. Thus, one may refer to silicone materials or zinc oxide–eugenol materials or even particular commercial brands of these materials.

A more general method of classification involves consideration of the properties of materials either before or after setting. Before setting, the property most normally used to characterize materials is viscosity. This may affect the fine detail which can be recorded in impressions of hard tissues and may influence the degree of tissue compression or displacement achieved with soft-tissue impressions. Thus, materials which are initially very fluid are

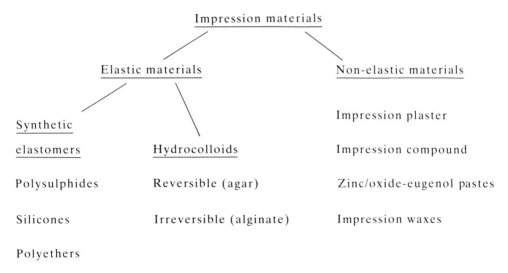

Fig. 16.1 Impression materials. Classified according to elastic properties and chemical type.

often classified as *mucostatic* impression materials because they are less likely to compress soft tissues, whilst materials which are initially more viscous are classified as *mucocompressive*. It should be remembered however, that viscosity often varies with the applied stress (p.17). Thus, certain materials which appear fairly viscous whilst under low stress conditions may become more fluid during the recording of the impression, when the material is placed under higher stress. When a substance behaves in this way, it is said to be *pseudoplastic*. Classification of materials according to viscosity is not, therefore, as simple as it may seem.

A more widely used classification of materials involves consideration of the properties of the set material. This factor is primarily responsible for governing the principal applications of the materials. The properties which are most important are *rigidity* and *elasticity*, since they determine whether an impression material can be used to record undercuts. When standing teeth are to be recorded, or when the patient has deep soft-tissue undercuts, the set impression material must be flexible enough to be withdrawn past the undercuts and elastic enough to give recovery and an accurate impression. Hence impression materials are classified as being *elastic* or *non-elastic*. The term 'elastic' as applied to impression materials is fairly unequivocal since the materials which form this group all possess the ability to be stretched or compressed and give a reasonable degree of elastic recovery following strain. The term 'non-elastic' however, is not a particularly good term with which to describe a group of products which in some cases are clearly plastic (e.g. impression waxes) and in other cases are very rigid but show little evidence of plastic deformation (e.g. impression plasters).

Fig. 16.1 lists the major groups of impression materials using the classification referred to above.

16.3 Requirements

The requirements of impression materials can be conveniently discussed under three main headings:

(1) Factors which affect the *accuracy* of the impression,

(2) Factors which affect the *dimensional stability* of the impression, that is, the way in which the accuracy varies with time after recording the impression,

(3) Manipulative variables such as ease of handling, setting characteristics etc.,

(4) Additional factors such as cost, taste, colour etc.

Accuracy

In order to record the fine detail of the hard or soft oral tissues, the impression material should be fluid on insertion into the patient's mouth. This requires a low viscosity or a degree of pseudoplasticity.

The way in which the material interacts with saliva is another factor affecting fine-detail reproduction. Some products are hydrophobic and may be repelled by moisture in a critical area of the impression. This normally results in the formation of a 'blow hole' in the impression. For such products, a dry field of operation is essential. Other materials are more compatible with moisture and saliva and no special precautions are necessary.

The 'setting' of impression materials, whether it involves a chemical reaction or simply a physical change of state, generally results in a dimensional change which, naturally, affects accuracy. For most materials, the dimensional change is a contraction and, providing the impression material is firmly attached to the impression tray, this produces an expansion of the impression 'space' and an oversized die, as illustrated in Fig. 16.2. Materials which expand during setting result in undersized dies or casts. The effect on the accuracy of fit of the resultant restoration depends on the type of restoration and the complexity of shape involved. For the simple crown preparation, illustrated in Fig. 16.2, the oversized die will result in a 'loose-fitting' crown. For greatest accuracy, the dimensional change should be minimal.

On being withdrawn from the patient's mouth, which is typically at a temperature of $32-37°C$, into

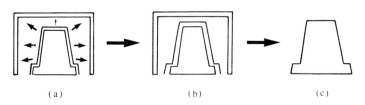

(a)   (b)   (c)

Fig. 16.2 Diagram illustrating the effect of setting contraction. (a) If the impression material is bonded to the tray, contraction occurs towards the tray. (b) Contraction results in an oversized impression space. (c) This results in an oversized die.

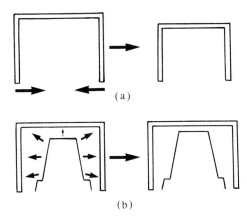

(a)

(b)

Fig. 16.3 Diagram illustrating the effects of thermal contraction. (a) The tray contracts and reduces the impression space. (b) The impression material contracts towards the tray (providing it is bonded) and increases the impression space.

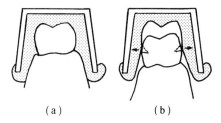

(a)   (b)

Fig. 16.4 Diagram illustrating how an impression material is placed under stress during removal from an undercut area. (a) Impression in place before removal. (b) During removal — the impression material is subjected to both compressive and tensile stresses.

the dental surgery, at a temperature of around 23°C, the impression undergoes approximately 10°C cooling. This results in thermal contraction, the magnitude of which depends on the value of coefficient of thermal expansion of the impression material and impression tray to which it is attached. It is difficult to calculate the precise value of the thermal contraction or to accurately predict the direction in which it operates since the contraction of the tray and that of the material act in opposite directions, providing the impression material remains attached to the tray. This is illustrated in Fig. 16.3. The effects of thermal changes are minimized if the values of coefficient of thermal expansion of the impression material and tray material are small.

It is important that the impression material remains attached to the impression tray during the recording of the impression. Partial detachment may cause gross distortions of the impression which may remain undetected and will almost certainly lead to ill-fitting appliances or restorations. Manufacturers of impression materials often supply tray adhesives which are used to enhance bonding. Additional retention is achieved by using perforated trays.

In addition to the requirements given above, there are two further requirements which apply specifically to materials used for recording undercuts. These materials must have adequate elastic properties and adequate tear resistance.

Fig. 16.4 shows diagramatically the way in which a set material is placed under stress during the withdrawal of the impression. The thickest parts of the impression are compressed against the tray when they pass the widest part of the tooth crown. As the impression is withdrawn it is likely that the material is also subjected to tensile stresses as the trapped material is stretched.

Fig. 16.5 gives a series of diagrams to illustrate what happens when an impression of an undercut tooth is recorded with (a) an elastic material, (b) a plastic material and (c) a viscoelastic material. The impression recorded with the elastic material accurately records the true shape of the tooth with

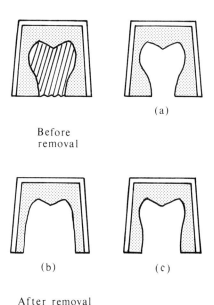

(a)

Before
removal

(b)   (c)

After removal

Fig. 16.5 Diagram illustrating attempts to record the impression of an undercut tooth crown with the following: (a) an elastic material; (b) a plastic material; (c) a viscoelastic material.

the correct degree of undercut. The impression recorded with the plastic material has been grossly distorted during removal and has not recorded any undercut. The impression recorded with the viscoelastic material gives a distorted shape. The degree of distortion depends on the severity of the undercut, the thickness of the impression material and the time for which the impression is maintained in a compressed state (Fig. 16.4b) as well as the viscoelastic properties of the material itself. The behaviour of viscoelastic materials is described on p. 15, where the influence of time as an important parameter is discussed in some detail. Ideally, an impression material used to record undercuts should be perfectly elastic. If a degree of viscoelasticity exists, distortions can be minimized by ensuring that the material is not maintained in the strained position for longer than necessary, by removing the impression quickly.

On removing elastic impression materials from undercut areas they are often put under a considerable tensile stress. The materials should be capable of withstanding such stresses without tearing. One important practical example of when tear resistance is required is shown in Fig. 16.6. For a crown preparation having subgingival shoulders, a thin, undercut region of impression material is formed. In order to obtain a complete impression this must not tear during removal of the impression.

Dimensional stability

The previous section deals with factors which affect the accuracy of an impression material during the periods of insertion into the patient's mouth, set-

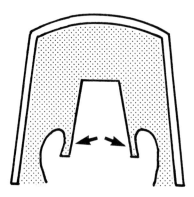

Fig. 16.6 Exaggerated view of a material being used to record an impression of a crown with subgingival shoulders. The thin areas of impression material, which are most prone to fracture, are arrowed.

ting, and withdrawal. The next stage is to cast a gypsum model into the impression. This stage is, however, often delayed for one of several reasons. It may not be convenient for the dentist himself to cast the model, in which case the impression is sent to a dental laboratory. If the laboratory is not on the same premises it may be several hours before the model is cast. If the laboratory is a long distance from the surgery it may be necessary to send the impression by post, in which case the delay between recording the impression and constructing the cast may be several days. The way in which the accuracy of the impression changes during this period is a measure of its dimensional stability. An ideal impression material would have perfect dimensional stability, such that the impression would retain its original accuracy indefinitely.

Several factors may contribute towards dimensional changes during storage or transportation of impressions. Continuation of the setting reaction beyond the apparent setting time may cause dimensional changes over a period of time. For viscoelastic materials, slow elastic recovery may continue for some time after withdrawal of the impression, producing a dimensional change. In this case the dimensional change results in a more accurate impression. For some 'elastic' materials it has been suggested that one should allow a rest period after withdrawing the impression, before pouring the gypsum cast, to allow elastic recovery to occur more fully. Some impression materials develop internal stresses on cooling from the temperature at which the impression is recorded to room temperature. This particularly applies to thermoplastic impression materials such as impression compound. On storage of the impression, distortions may occur as the material attempts to relieve the internal stresses. Finally, many impression materials contain volatile substances, either as primary components or as byproducts of the setting reactions. Loss of such volatile materials during storage results in a shrinkage of the impression material with a consequent decrease in accuracy. For the majority of materials, accuracy is best maintained by pouring the gypsum cast soon after recording the impression.

Manipulative variables

Many methods of dispensation are used for impression materials. Some involve the mixing of powder and water, others paste and liquid, others two

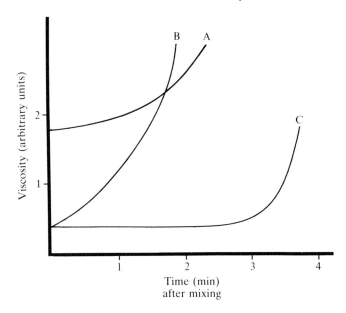

Fig. 16.7 Viscosity versus time curves for three impression materials. Material A is initially quite viscous and its viscosity slowly increases. Material B is initially fluid (low viscosity) but its viscosity increases sharply. Material C is initially fluid and has an induction period during which viscosity is constant. This is followed by a rapid increase in viscosity.

pastes and some require no mixing at all. The latter materials, generally, require warming in either a water bath or bunsen flame in order to soften them. They record the impression by rehardening at mouth temperature. For materials where mixing is required, the two-paste systems, generally supplied in toothpaste-like tubes, have certain advantages. Proportioning is easy; one simply 'squeezes' out equal lengths of paste from each tube onto a paper mixing pad or a glass plate. The manufacturer normally supplies the two pastes with contrasting colours so that it is easy to see when mixing has been completed satisfactorily — there are no streaks of colour left in the mix. For powder/liquid and paste/liquid systems, it is not possible to define clearly the point at which mixing has been completed satisfactorily. If mixing is incomplete, certain parts of the impression may remain unset.

The setting characteristics of the material have an important effect on the ease of handling and, therefore, often influence the dental surgeon's choice of product. Materials which soften on warming and 'set' on cooling are sometimes difficult to control, particularly in inexperienced hands. The setting characteristics are almost totally under the control of the operator since they depend on the temperature to which the material is heated and the time for which it is maintained at that temperature before recording the impression.

For those materials which set by a chemical reaction, setting begins immediately after mixing unless the manufacturer incorporates a retarder.

The *working time* of the material is the time, from start of mix, until the material is no longer suitable for recording an impression. It is normally characterized by the time taken for the viscosity to increase by a given amount above that of the freshly mixed material. Several methods are available for measuring the increase in viscosity as a function of time, including cone and plate viscometers, extrusion rheometers, reciprocating rheometers and simple parallel-plate plastimeters. In each case, the value of working time obtained is somewhat arbitrary, since it depends on a subjective decision as to the degree of increase in viscosity which can be tolerated before the material becomes unworkable. Three typical viscosity–time curves for impression materials are given in Fig. 16.7. Curve A represents a material for which viscosity is high immediately after mixing but increases relatively slowly over the first three minutes. Curve B represents a material, the initial viscosity of which is low but increases rapidly after mixing. Curve C represents a material for which viscosity remains constant for some time due to retardation of the setting reaction. Following the induction period, the viscosity increases rapidly. With materials which do not have an induction period the impression should be recorded as soon as possible after mixing to ensure that the viscosity has not increased unduly.

Whereas the working times of materials are determined at room temperature, setting times are generally determined at mouth temperature. The *setting time* of an impression material may be defined in terms of the time required to complete the setting reaction. It is more normal, however, to use a definition which is based on the time to reach a certain degree of rigidity, hardness or elasticity. Setting times measured in this way often give values which are significantly shorter than the times required to complete the setting reaction, indicating that setting continues slowly for some time after removal from the mouth. In order to obtain the optimum performance from any impression material, it is wise to leave the material in the patient's mouth for an extra minute or so after setting has apparently been completed. This particularly applies to the elastic materials for which significant improvements in elasticity may occur after the apparent completion of setting.

For the convenience and comfort of both the dental surgeon and patient the most ideal combination of properties for an impression material is a long working time and short setting time. This can be achieved with materials which set by a chemical reaction providing the reaction rate is much quicker at mouth temperature than at room temperature.

Additional requirements
An impression material should be non-toxic, non-irritant, clean to use and have an acceptable odour and taste. It should also have a long shelf life so that unused material can be stored without deteriorating and should be relatively cheap if it is to gain wide acceptance.

17 Non-elastic Impression Materials

17.1 Introduction

Four main types of products form the group of impression materials classified as non-elastic materials. These are:

(1) Impression plaster,
(2) Impression compound,
(3) Impression waxes,
(4) Zinc oxide/eugenol impression pastes.

They are classified together for convenience rather than for reasons of similarity in composition or properties. A factor which links the materials is their inability to accurately record undercuts. One of the materials (plaster) is brittle when set and fractures when withdrawn over undercuts. The other products are likely to undergo gross distortions due to plastic flow if used in undercut situations.

17.2 Impression plaster

Impression plaster is similar in composition to the dental plaster used to construct models and dies (Chap. 3). It consists of calcined, β-calcium sulphate hemihydrate which when mixed with water reacts to form calcium sulphate dihydrate.

The material is used at a higher water/powder ratio (approximately 0·60) than is normally used for modelling plasters. The fluid mix is required to enable fine detail to be recorded in the impression and to give the material *mucostatic* properties. The setting expansion of dental plaster is reduced to minimal proportions by using *anti-expansion agents*. Potassium sulphate is the most common of these and has the secondary effect of accelerating the setting reaction, details of which are discussed on p. 27. A retarder, such as borax, is normally incorporated, in order to give a material in which the setting characteristics are controlled. A pigment such as alazarin red is also commonly used, in order to make a clear distinction between the impression and the model after casting of the model.

The anti-expansion agent, retarder and pigment are incorporated into the impression plaster powder by some manufacturers. As an alternative an *anti-expansion solution*, containing potassium sulphate, borax and pigment, may be prepared and used with a standard white plaster.

Freshly mixed plaster is too fluid to be used in a stock impression tray and is normally used in a special tray, constructed using a 1–1·5 mm spacer. The tray may be constructed from acrylic resin or shellac. Another technique is to record the plaster impression as a wash in a preliminary compound impression. The compound is deliberately moved during setting to create space for the plaster wash.

Before casting a plaster model in a plaster impression, the impression must be coated with a separating agent, otherwise separation is impossible.

The mixed impression material is initially very fluid and is capable of recording soft tissues in the uncompressed state. In addition, the hemihydrate particles are capable of absorbing moisture from the surface of the oral soft tissues, allowing very intimate contact between the impression material and the tissues. The fluidity of the material, combined with the ability to remove moisture from tissues and a minimal dimensional change on setting, results in a very accurate impression which may be difficult to remove.

The water-absorbing nature of these materials often causes patients to complain about a very dry sensation after having impressions recorded.

Following setting, the plaster impression material is very brittle. It can undergo virtually no compressive or tensile strain without fracturing. The material is, therefore, not suitable for use in any undercut situations. One technique for recording impressions of undercut areas, commonly used before the advent of elastic materials, was to allow the impression plaster to 'set' and then to fracture it in order to facilitate removal from the mouth. The material is weak and easily fractured due to its high water/powder radio. The fragments are then reconstructed in order to form the completed impression.

17.3 Impression compound

Impression compound is a thermoplastic material, having properties which in many ways are similar to those of the dental waxes discussed in Chap. 4. The composition varies from one product to another but an indication of typical composition is given in Table 17.1. Two types of impression compound are available. These are usually classified as type I (lower fusing) and type II (higher fusing). The type I materials are impression materials whereas the type II materials are used for constructing impression trays. The difference in fusing temperature between type I and type II materials naturally reflects a difference in the composition of the thermoplastic components of each.

The lower fusing, type I impression materials may be supplied in either sheet or stick form. The sheet material is used for recording impressions of edentulous ridges, normally using stock trays. The stick material is used for border extensions on impression trays or for recording impressions of single crowns using the *copper ring* technique.

The sheet material is normally softened using a water bath. Both the temperature and time of conditioning in the water bath affect the performance of the material. If the conditioning temperature is too low, the material does not soften properly, and if too high, it becomes sticky and unmanageable. A temperature in the range 55–60°C is normally found to be ideal.

The conditioning time must also be carefully monitored. It should not be so long that important constituents, such as stearic acid, can be leached out, nor should it be so short that the material is not thoroughly softened. The materials are poor conductors of heat and it may take several minutes for the centre of the material to become softened.

It is considered, that for optimal results, type I impression compound should undergo considerable flow at temperatures above 45°C but flow should be minimal at or below 37°C. The stick material is generally softened using a bunsen burner. A measure of skill and experience is required in order to soften the material sufficiently without causing it to become too fluid or to ignite. The material is tempered in a water bath before placing in the patient's mouth.

The copper ring technique involves the recording of single crown preparations in stick compound employing a hollow, open-ended copper tube as a type of 'tray'. The principle is illustrated in Fig. 17.1.

Impression compound is the most viscous of the impression materials in common use. Table 17.2 gives typical values of viscosity for some materials, measured at a given shear rate. It can be seen that under these conditions the viscosity is some 70 times greater than that for impression plaster and more than 100 times greater than values for some of the light-bodied elastomers. The very high viscosity of impression compound is significant in two ways. Firstly, it limits the degree of fine detail which can be recorded in an impression. Secondly, it characterizes compound as a mucocompressive impression material. In certain circumstances, the high viscosity is used to advantage. For example, when recording impressions of some edentulous patients it is necessary to record the full depth of the sulcus so that a denture with adequate retention can be designed. Only a viscous material, such as compound, is able to displace the lingual and buccal soft tissues sufficiently.

Compound is fairly rigid after setting and has poor elastic properties. A large stress would be required to remove an impression from undercut areas and the resultant impression would be grossly distorted. The materials have large values of coefficient of thermal expansion and undergo consider-

Table 17.1 Composition of a typical impression compound material

Component	Example	Function
Thermoplastic material (47 percent)	Natural or synthetic resins and waxes	Characterizes the softening temperature.
Filler (50 percent)	Talc	Gives 'body' by increasing viscosity of the softened material. Reduces thermal contraction.
Lubricant (3 percent)	Stearic acid	Improves flow properties.

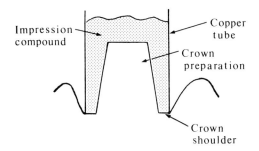

Fig. 17.1 Diagram illustrating the principle of the copper ring technique for obtaining impressions of crown preparations.

Table 17.2 Viscosity values for some impression materials*

Material	Viscosity (Pas)
Impression compound	4000
Impression plaster	60
Zinc oxide/eugenol paste	60
Alginate	50
Light-bodied elastomer	30
'Putty' elastomer	800

*Measured at 50 s⁻¹ shear rate and 1 minute after mixing — for materials which require mixing.

able shrinkage on removal from the mouth. This can be partially overcome by resoftening the surface of the impression with a bunsen flame and reseating the impression.

Three factors combine to produce significant internal stresses within the compound impression. These are:

(1) The high value of coefficient of thermal expansion,

(2) The poor thermal conductivity,

(3) The relatively large temperature drop from the softening temperature to room temperature.

The gradual relief of internal stresses may cause distortion of the impression. For the most accurate results, the model should be poured as soon as possible after recording the impression.

Impression compound is most widely used for recording preliminary impressions of edentulous arches. The high viscosity of the material enables the full depth of the sulcus to be recorded. This gives a model on which a special tray can be constructed. A major impression is recorded in the special tray using a less viscous material, such as zinc oxide/eugenol impression paste.

17.4 Impression waxes

Impression waxes are rarely used to record complete impressions but are normally used to correct small imperfections in other impressions, particularly those of the zinc oxide/eugenol type. They may also be used to record impressions of free-end saddles in certain techniques. They are thermoplastic materials which flow readily at mouth temperature and are relatively soft even at room temperature. They are used in small quantities to 'fill in' areas of impressions in which insufficient material has been used or in which an 'air blow' has caused a defect.

These materials consist, typically, of a mixture of a low melting paraffin wax and beeswax in a ratio of about 3:1. This composition ensures a very high degree of flow at mouth temperature.

17.5 Zinc oxide/eugenol impression pastes

These materials are normally supplied as two pastes which are mixed together on a paper pad or glass slab. Typical compositions of the two pastes are given in Table 17.3. There is normally a good colour contrast between the two pastes, the zinc oxide paste, typically, being white and the eugenol paste, a reddish brown colour. This enables thorough mixing to be achieved as indicated by a homogeneous colour, free of streaks, in the mixed material.

The pastes are normally dispensed from toothpaste-like tubes and are mixed in equal volumes. The proportioning is achieved, simply, by expressing equal lengths of each paste onto the mixing pad or slab. The manufacturers normally label one of the tubes as the catalyst paste and the other the base paste. Some manufacturers refer to the zinc oxide paste as the catalyst paste, whilst others refer to it as the base paste.

On mixing the two pastes, a reaction between zinc oxide and eugenol begins. Fig. 17.2 gives the structural formula of eugenol. The basis of the reaction is that the phenolic $-OH$ of the eugenol acts as a weak acid and undergoes an acid−base reaction with zinc oxide to form a salt, zinc eugenolate, as follows:

$$2C_{10}H_{12}O_2 + ZnO \rightarrow Zn(C_{10}H_{11}O_2)_2 + H_2O$$

Two molecules of eugenol react with zinc oxide to form the salt. The structural formula of zinc eugenolate is given in Fig. 17.3. It can be seen that

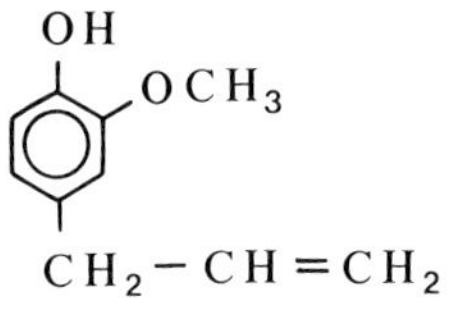

OH
OCH₃

CH₂−CH=CH₂

Fig. 17.2 Structural formula of eugenol.

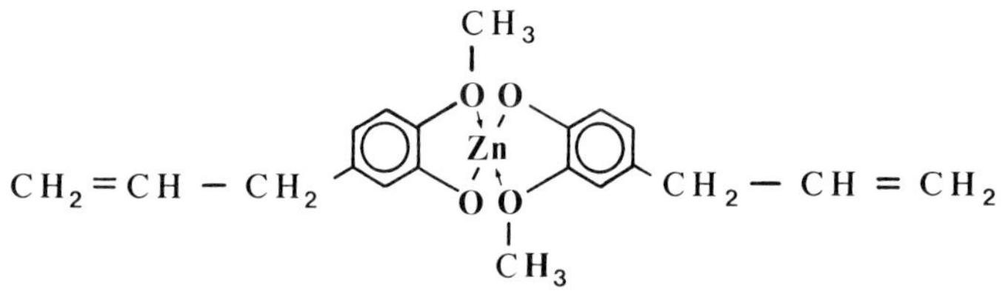

CH₃
O O
Zn
CH₂=CH − CH₂   CH₂− CH = CH₂
O O
CH₃

Fig. 17.3 Structural formula of zinc eugenolate.

Table 17.3 Composition of zinc oxide/eugenol impression pastes

	Component	Function
Paste 1	Zinc oxide	Reactive ingredient which takes part in setting reaction.
	Olive oil, linseed oil or equivalent	Inert component used to form paste with zinc oxide.
	Zinc acetate or equivalent (in small quantities)	To accelerate setting.
	Water (trace) in some products	To accelerate setting.
Paste 2	Eugenol (oil of cloves)	Reactive ingredient — takes part in setting reaction.
	Kaolin, talc or equivalent	Inert filler used to form a paste with eugenol.

the ionic salt bonds are formed between zinc and the phenolic oxygens of each molecule of eugenol. Two further co-ordinate bonds are formed by donation of pairs of electrons from the methoxy oxygens to zinc. These bonds are indicated by the arrows in Fig. 17.3. Although the structural formula shows the two aromatic rings lying in the plane of the paper, in fact, they occupy perpendicular planes, such that one ring is in the plane of the paper whilst the other is in a plane at 90° to the plane of the paper. The structure can, therefore, be visualized as a central zinc atom held by two eugenol 'claws'. Compounds with this type of structure are normally referred to as *chelate compounds*.

The setting reaction is ionic in nature and re-

quires an ionic medium in which to proceed at any pace. The ionic nature is increased by the presence of water and certain ionizable salts which act as accelerators. Some manufacturers do not incorporate water into the pastes and for these materials setting is retarded until the mixed paste contacts moisture in the patient's mouth. Water is then absorbed and setting is accelerated. Other manufacturers include water as a component of at least one of the pastes, in order that setting can commence immediately after mixing.

These materials are normally used to record the major impressions of edentulous arches. The impression is normally recorded in a close-fitting special tray, constructed on the model obtained from the primary impression, or inside the patient's existing denture.

The thickness of paste used is normally around 1 mm. This thin section of material results in an insignificant dimensional change on setting and subsequent storage of the impression. The relatively low initial viscosity of the mixed paste, coupled with its pseudoplastic nature, allows fine detail to be recorded in the impression. Defects sometimes arise on the surface of the impression but these can be corrected using an impression wax.

The major restriction on the use of these materials is their lack of elasticity. The set material distorts or fractures when removed over undercuts.

For the vast majority of patients the zinc oxide/eugenol impression pastes may be considered non-irritant. Occasionally, however, eugenol may promote an allergic response in some patients. To cater for this type of patient, eugenol-free zinc oxide impression pastes are available. The eugenol is replaced by an alternative organic acid.

18   Elastic Impression Materials — Hydrocolloids

18.1 Introduction

Hydrocolloid impression materials used in dentistry are based on colloidal suspensions of polysaccharides in water. A colloidal suspension is characterized by the fact that it behaves neither as a solution, in which the solute is dissolved in the solvent, nor as a true suspension, in which a heterogeneous structure exists with solid particles being suspended in a liquid. The colloidal suspension lies somewhere between these two extremes; no solid particles can be detected and yet the mixture does not behave as a simple solution. When the fluid medium of the colloid is water it is normally referred to as a hydrocolloid.

Dental hydrocolloid impression materials exist in two forms: sol or gel form. In the sol form, they are fluid with low viscosity and there is a random arrangement of the polysaccharide chains. In the gel form, the materials are more viscous and may develop elastic properties if the long polysaccharide chains become aligned.

The conversion from sol to gel forms the basis of the setting of the hydrocolloid impression materials. The products are introduced into the patient's mouth while in the fluid, sol form. When conversion to gel is complete, and elastic properties have been developed, the impression is removed and the model cast.

The formation of gel and development of elastic properties through alignment of polysaccharide chains may take place by one of two mechanisms. For some materials, gel formation is induced by cooling the sol. Chains become aligned and are mutually attracted by Van der Waals forces. Intermolecular hydrogen bonds may be formed between adjacent chains, enhancing the elasticity of the gel. On reheating the gel, these bonds are readily destroyed and the material reverts to the sol form. These materials are the *reversible hydrocolloids* (agar). The principle of gel formation is given in Fig. 18.1.

For other materials, gel formation involves the production of strong intermolecular cross-links between polysaccharide chains. These materials do not require cooling in order to encourage gel formation and once formed the gel does not readily revert to the sol form. These materials are the *irreversible hydrocolloids* (alginates).

18.2 Reversible hydrocolloids (agar)

These materials are normally supplied as a gel in a flexible, toothpaste-like tube. The gel consists primarily of a 15 percent colloidal suspension of agar in water. Agar is a complex polysaccharide which is extracted from seaweed. Fig. 18.2 gives a very simplified indication of the type of molecular structure. The high molecular weight, coupled with the large concentration of free hydroxyl groups, renders the material suitable for hydrocolloid formation.

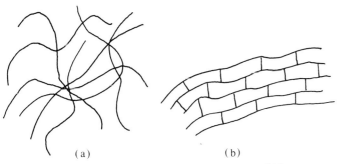

Fig. 18.1 Diagram illustrating the formation of an aqueous polysaccharide gel by ordering of the polymer chains. (a) Disordered chains (present in sol). (b) Ordered chains (present in gel). Chemical cross-links are formed in irreversible materials.

(a)   (b)

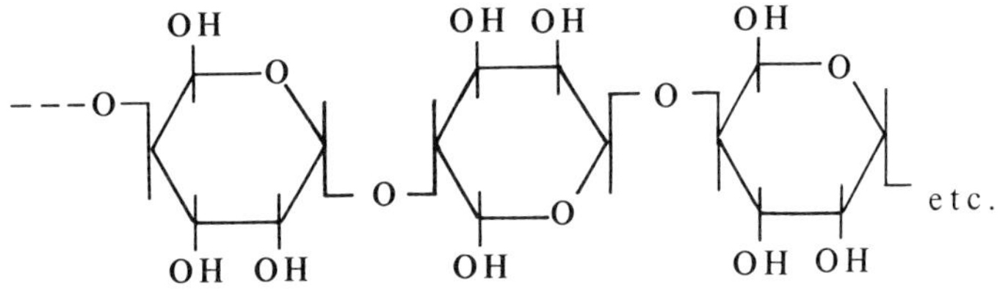

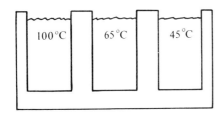

Fig. 18.2 Simplified structural formula of a polysaccharide chain similar to that used in agar.

Fig. 18.3 A specialized water bath used for conditioning agar impression material.

Small quantities of borax and potassium sulphate are normally present in the gel. Borax is added to give more 'body' to the gel, although the mechanism by which this is achieved is unclear. Unfortunately, borax retards the setting of gypsum model and die materials and models formed in agar impressions may have surfaces of poor quality. The presence of potassium sulphate in the agar gel counteracts this effect of the borax, since it accelerates the setting of gypsum products. (See p. 30.)

Manipulation Reversible hydrocolloids are normally conditioned, prior to use, using a specially designed conditioning bath. This consists of three compartments each containing water (Fig. 18.3).

The tube of gel is first placed in the 100°C bath. This rapidly converts the gel to sol and the contents of the tube become very fluid. The tube is then transferred to the 65°C bath where it is stored until required for use. This temperature is high enough to maintain the material in the sol form. At this stage, the material is mixed by squeezing the tube, thus ensuring an even distribution of components. A few minutes before the impression is recorded, the contents are cooled to 45°C. If the material is maintained at this temperature for long, it slowly begins to revert to the gel form. When the impression is recorded, the sol is expressed from the tube into an impression tray and seated in the patient's mouth. The conversion from sol to gel takes place slowly at mouth temperature and it may be many minutes before the material develops sufficient elasticity to permit removal of the impression. The rate of conversion of sol to gel may be accelerated by spraying cold water onto the impression tray whilst it is in the mouth, or by using water-cooled impression trays. The latter are metal trays with a narrow-bore metal tube attached to the outer surface. The tube is connected to a cold water supply and the circulating water reduces the temperature of the tray. The coolest areas of the sol are converted to gel more rapidly, so the material in contact with the tray sets more rapidly than that in contact with the oral tissues. It is argued that this arrangement may be advantageous. If slight movements of the impression tray take place during setting, the material adjacent to the oral tissues can flow to compensate, thus reducing inaccuracies.

After preparation of the model, the material can be re-used, as it is readily converted to sol by reheating and can be sterilized before use on another patient.

Properties In the sol form, agar is sufficiently fluid to allow detailed reproduction of hard and soft oral tissues. Its low viscosity classifies it as a mucostatic material, as it does not compress or displace soft tissues.

In the gel form, agar is sufficiently flexible to be withdrawn past undercuts. The materials are viscoelastic and the elastic recovery can be optimized by using correct technique. A suitable model used to explain the nature of viscoelastic materials is described on p. 14. (Refer to Fig. 2.15.) The amount of permanent deformation exhibited by a viscoelastic impression material is a function of the severity of the undercuts and the time for which the material is under stress during the removal of the impression. The elastic recovery is enhanced and permanent deformation reduced if the impression is removed in one quick movement, ensuring that the impression material is under stress only momentarily.

Agar gel has very poor mechanical properties and tears at very low levels of stress. Interproximal

Table 18.1 Composition of alginate impression material powders

Material	Function
Sodium or potassium salt of alginic acid	Main reactive ingredient. Forms sol with water and becomes cross-linked to form gel.
$CaSO_4 \cdot 2H_2O$ (gypsum)	Source of Ca^{2+} ions which cause cross-linking of the alginate chains.
Na_3PO_4	Used to control the working time.
Inert filler — such as diatomaceous earth	Gives 'body' and enables easy manipulation.
Reaction indicator (present in some products)	Gives a colour change when setting is complete.

and subgingival areas are very difficult to record with this type of impression material.

The material has very poor dimensional stability — a function of the very high water content of the gel. On standing, water is readily lost by a combination of syneresis and evaporation. The process of *syneresis* may be envisaged as a squeezing out of water from between polysaccharide chains. As a result, one can often observe small droplets of water on the surface of an agar impression. The water may be lost by evaporation, causing shrinkage of the impression and seriously affecting accuracy. In the presence of excess water, agar gel may absorb water by a process which is, effectively, the reverse of syneresis. This process is referred to as *imbibition*. When water is imbibed it causes a separation of the aligned polysaccharide chains and a swelling of the impression. In order to assure optimum accuracy the model should be cast as soon as possible.

The primary uses of agar impressions are for partial denture and crown and bridge patients. For these applications, the poor tear resistance is considered to be their major disadvantage.

18.3 Irreversible hydrocolloids (alginates)

Alginate impression materials are supplied as powders which are mixed with water. The typical composition of an alginate powder is given in Table 18.1. The relative concentration of each ingredient varies from one product to another. Some alginates are more fluid than others because they contain less

filler, while some products are faster setting than others because they contain less trisodium phosphate.

Manipulation The normal method of dispensing the materials is in large tubs. Scoops are provided for measuring the powder whilst plastic measuring cylinders are generally used to meter the correct volume of water. An alternative method of dispensation is to supply the alginate powder in small sachets. The contents of one sachet are sufficient for one impression. The operator simply adds the correct volume of water. This ensures a correct concentration of ingredients in each impression. Materials supplied in tubs have a tendency to undergo separation as the dense ingredients fall to the bottom of the container. This must be overcome by inverting the container before use. It also prevents compaction of the powder and ensures that a reproducible volume of material is used in each mix. After proportioning, the powder and water are mixed together in a plastic mixing bowl using a wide-bladed spatula. Rapid spatulation is required to give thorough mixing and an alginate sol of 'creamy' consistency. The material is used in either stock trays or special trays and an adhesive is used to aid retention of the impression material by the tray.

Setting reaction On mixing and spatulating the powder and water, an alginate sol is formed. The sodium phosphate, present in the powder, dissolves readily in the water whilst the gypsum is only sparingly soluble (solubility about 0·2 percent).

The structural formula of sodium alginate is given in Fig. 18.4a. This may be represented by the simplified structure given in Fig. 18.4b for the purpose of clarifying the setting reaction.

Sodium alginate readily reacts with calcium ions derived from the dissolved gypsum to form calcium alginate, as shown in Fig. 18.5. The replacement of monovalent sodium with divalent calcium results in the cross-linking of the alginate chains and the conversion of the material from the sol to gel form. As the setting reaction proceeds, and the degree of cross-linking increases, the gel develops elastic properties.

Sodium phosphate plays an important role in controlling the setting characteristics of alginate materials. It reacts rapidly with calcium ions as they are formed giving insoluble calcium phosphate.

$$3Ca^{2+} + 2Na_3PO_4 \rightarrow Ca_3(PO_4)_2 + 6Na^+$$

This reaction denies the supply of calcium ions

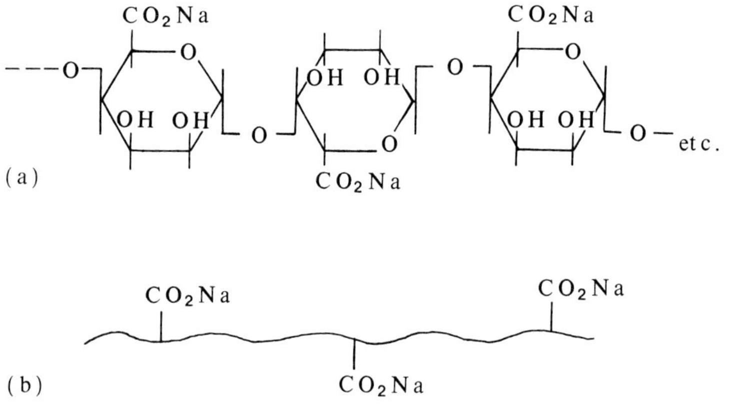

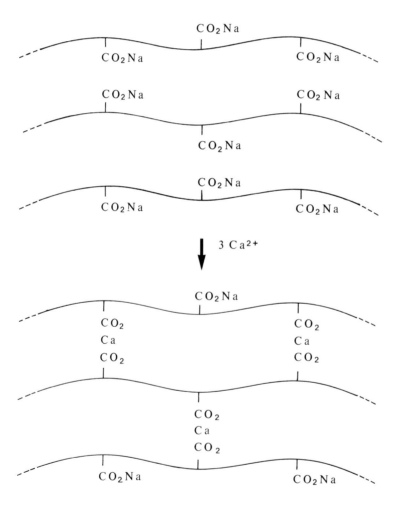

(a)

(b)

Fig. 18.4 The structural formula of sodium alginate. (a) Actual formula. (b) Simplified formula.

$3\ Ca^{2+}$

Fig. 18.5 Schematic representation of the cross-linking of alginate chains by replacement of sodium ions with calcium ions.

required to complete the cross-linking of alginate chains and thus extends the working time of the material. When all the sodium phosphate has reacted, calcium ions become available for reaction with sodium alginate, the setting reaction is initiated and the viscosity of the material increases rapidly.

Properties The freshly spatulated material has low viscosity (Table 17.2), although this can be varied to some extent by alterations in the amount of inert filler incorporated by the manufacturer. The low viscosity, coupled with a degree of pseudo-plasticity, classifies alginates as mucostatic impression materials. They are able to record soft tissues in the uncompressed state. For some applications low viscosity may be a disadvantage, for example, when trying to record the depth of the lingual sulcus. A higher viscosity is required to displace the lingual soft tissues in order that the full depth can be recorded.

It follows from the description of the setting reaction that these products go through an induction period following mixing, during which the viscosity remains almost unaltered. This is followed by rapid setting. The setting characteristics of these materials, therefore, approach the ideal requirement of adequate working time followed by rapid setting. They are unique from this point of view. The setting characteristics can be further controlled by the operator by fixing the temperature of the water used. The use of warm water reduces the working time and setting time both by accelerating the rate at which sodium phosphate is consumed and by subsequently increasing the rate of the cross-linking reaction. The use of cold water, naturally, has the reverse effect.

In contrast to the reversible hydrocolloids, alginate material adjacent to the oral tissues sets more rapidly, while that adjacent to the cooler tray wall sets more slowly. Hence, the operator must ensure that the impression tray is not moved during setting, otherwise distortions occur.

Following setting, the material is flexible and elastic enough to be withdrawn past undercuts, although it should be remembered that, as for agar, the alginate materials are viscoelastic and due regard to this should be made when withdrawing the impression from the patient's mouth (see Section 18.2). The degree of cross-linking continues to increase after the material has apparently set. Waiting a further minute or two before removing

the impression enhances the elastic nature of the materials.

Alginate gels have poor mechanical properties and are liable to tear when removed from deep undercuts, particularly in interproximal and sub-gingival areas.

Permanent distortions due to viscoelastic effects and tearing are reduced slightly by using a large bulk of material. It is normal to have approximately 5 mm of material between the tissues and the tray.

The model should be cast as soon as possible, in order to prevent inaccuracies due to dimensional changes, because alginate impressions undergo syneresis and imbibition by the same mechanisms described for agar (Section 18.2). The impressions may be stored for a short time if covered with a damp napkin.

Alginate impression materials are widely used for a variety of applications. In prosthodontics, they are used for recording impressions of edentulous and partially edentulous arches. In orthodontics, they are used for recording impressions prior to appliance construction and they are used extensively for recording impressions for study model construction. They are only rarely used for crown and bridge work because their poor tear resistance is a serious disadvantage when considering this application.

18.4 Modified alginates

Alginates modified by the incorporation of silicone polymers have been developed. These are supplied as two pastes which are mixed together. A colour contrast between the pastes enables thorough mixing to be achieved although this can be difficult because the pastes are of widely differing viscosity in some products.

The setting characteristics of the modified alginate materials are similar to those of the conventional products. They show marginally better fine-detail reproduction and tear resistance but have poor dimensional stability. They lose water at about the same rate as a conventional alginate if allowed to stand. Casts should be poured soon after recording impressions if accuracy is to be maintained.

The materials are considered as hybrids of alginates and silicone elastomers but their properties are closely related to those of the alginates.

19 Elastic Impression Materials — Synthetic Elastomers

19.1 Introduction

Synthetic elastomers were developed mainly for industrial applications but their potential in medicine and dentistry was quickly realized and they are now widely used as impression materials. They were quick to gain acceptance in dentistry because they offered potential solutions to the two main problems associated with hydrocolloids — poor tear resistance and poor dimensional stability.

Four types of elastomers are in general use. These are:

(1) Polysulphides,
(2) Silicone rubbers, (condensation curing type),
(3) Silicone rubbers (addition curing type),
(4) Polyethers.

19.2 Polysulphides

Composition These materials are generally supplied as two pastes which are dispensed from tubes. One paste is normally labelled base paste whilst the other is labelled catalyst paste. The composition of a typical material is given in Table 19.1.

The liquid polysulphide prepolymer in the base paste is of complex structure but, for mechanistic purposes, it may be represented by the simplified structure given in Fig. 19.1. The viscosity of the paste is governed by the quantity of filler incorporated by the manufacturer. Three grades of paste are normally available to the practitioner — 'light-bodied', 'regular-bodied' and 'heavy-bodied', having increasing filler contents and viscosity values.

The base paste is normally white, due to the filler, and has an unpleasant odour caused by the high concentration of thiol groups. The colour of the catalyst paste is governed by the nature of the oxidizing agent used; materials containing lead dioxide are normally dark brown. The colour contrast between the two pastes is an aid to efficient

Table 19.1 Composition of polysulphide impression materials

	Component	Function
Base paste	Polysulphide prepolymer with terminal and pendant thiol (−SH) groups	This is further polymerized and cross-linked to form rubber.
	Inert filler — possibly chalk or titanium dioxide	To give 'body', control viscosity and modify physical properties.
Catalyst paste	Lead dioxide or other alternative oxidizing agent	To react with thiol groups — causing setting.
	Sulphur	Involved in setting reaction.
	Inert oil — normally paraffinic type	To form a paste with PbO_2 and sulphur.

mixing, which is continued until a homogeneous colour, with no streaks, is achieved. An adhesive is used to promote adhesion between the impression material and tray.

Setting reaction On mixing the two pastes, terminal and pendant thiol groups of the prepolymer chains undergo a reaction with lead dioxide. Some of these reactions result in chain extension and cross-linking as shown in Fig. 19.2. The reaction is of the *condensation polymerization* type since one molecule of water is produced as a byproduct of each reaction stage. As chain extension proceeds, the viscosity increases. When the degree of cross-linking reaches a certain level the material develops elastic properties.

Properties The setting characteristics of the polysulphides differ considerably from those of the

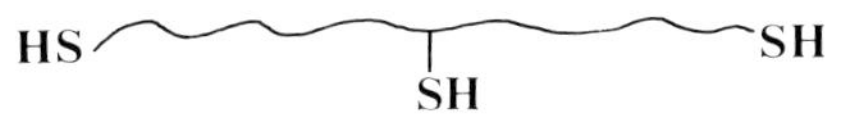

HS ⌇⌇⌇⌇⌇⌇⌇⌇ SH
        |
        SH

Fig 19.1 Simplified structural formula of the polysulphide prepolymer showing terminal and pendant −SH groups.

alginates (p. 115). Setting commences immediately on mixing of the two pastes and is characterized by a gradual increase in viscosity and a rather slow development of elasticity. Setting times of ten minutes or more are not uncommon, particularly for light-bodied materials. The polysulphide elastomers have very good tear resistance. They can, typically, withstand about 700 percent tensile strain before tearing. Some of this strain is non-recoverable, since the elastic properties of these materials are far from ideal. They are considered as viscoelastic and recover only slowly and not completely after being compressed or stretched. The time required for recovery and the degree of permanent deformation are functions of the severity of the undercuts and the time during which the material is under strain. In order to optimize elastic recovery the impression should be removed with a single, swift pull.

Many of the properties of these products are directly related to the amount of filler incorporated in the pastes. This particularly applies to viscosity, setting contraction, thermal contraction after removal of the impression from the mouth and dimensional stability (Table 19.2). It can be seen that the heavy-bodied materials are potentially more accurate, since they exhibit less setting and thermal contraction and have better dimensional stability. Their high viscosity means that they are unable to record the same level of fine detail as the more fluid, light-bodied materials.

Dimensional changes occuring after apparent setting of polysulphides are due to two major factors. Firstly, continued reaction occurs for some time after the apparent setting time, causing further shrinkage. Secondly, water produced as a byproduct of the setting reaction may be lost by evaporation from the surface. In this case the dimensional change is also associated with a change in weight of the material. The better dimensional stability of the heavy-bodied materials is due to the fact that they contain a lower concentration of reactive groups and therefore produce fewer byproducts. Although the polysulphides do not have perfect dimensional stability they perform far better than hydrocolloids in this respect.

The use of lead compounds in polysulphide materials has been questioned because of the known toxic effects of lead. It is unlikely that the lead contained in these products is able to exert a harmful effect as the material is in the patient's mouth for only a few minutes and is hydrophobic, reducing the chances of 'washing-out' of lead compounds by saliva. The use of lead-free polysulphides is likely to increase, however, as a wider range of alternative materials becomes available.

Applications Polysulphides are commonly used for crown and bridge impressions and only infrequently for other applications. In order to fabricate restorations which have a good fit, it is important that the impression be as accurate as possible. This is generally achieved by using special trays and either a regular-bodied material or a heavy-bodied and light-bodied material in combination. There are many variations on the latter technique. One commonly used method is to load a syringe with freshly mixed light-bodied material and the impres-

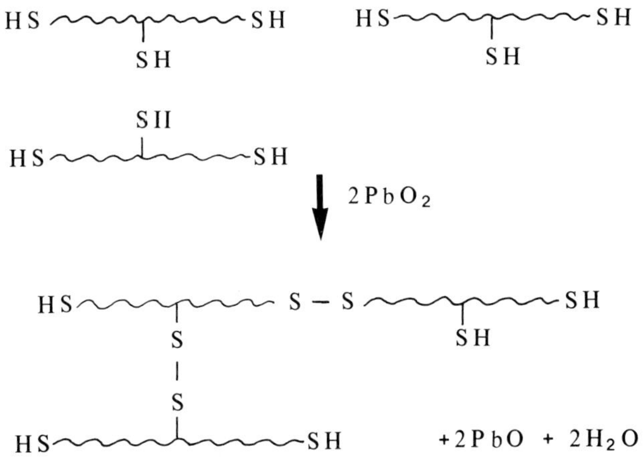

HS ⌇⌇⌇⌇⌇ SH   HS ⌇⌇⌇⌇⌇ SH
        | |
        SH   SH

        S H
         |
HS ⌇⌇⌇⌇⌇ SH

        ↓ $2 PbO_2$

HS ⌇⌇⌇⌇ S − S ⌇⌇⌇⌇ SH
        | |
        S   SH
        |
        S
        |
HS ⌇⌇⌇⌇ SH $+ 2 PbO + 2 H_2O$

Fig. 19.2 Schematic representation of the chain lengthening and cross-linking of the polysulphide prepolymer through oxidation of the −SH groups forming disulphide links. Water is liberated as a byproduct.

Table 19.2 Influence of filler content on some properties of polysulphides

Filler content	Light-bodied	Viscosity	Setting contraction	Thermal contraction	Dimensional stability
|	Regular-bodied	|	|	|	|
Increasing		Increasing	Decreasing	Decreasing	Increasing
↓	Heavy-bodied	↓	↓	↓	↓

sion tray with freshly mixed heavy-bodied material. The light-bodied material is injected around those teeth on which cavities have been cut or crown cores prepared. The tray, containing heavy-bodied material, is then seated so that the two materials can set simultaneously. Fig. 19.3 is a line diagram which gives the appearance of the impression viewed in cross-section. It can be seen that the bulk of the impression is recorded in heavy-bodied material — assuring optimum accuracy and dimensional stability. The thin layer of the impression adjacent to the oral tissues is recorded in light-bodied material — assuring optimum fine-detail reproduction.

A variation on the above technique is a two-stage method in which an initial impression is recorded in heavy-bodied material. The impression is reseated, with a small quantity of freshly mixed light-bodied material in the area of interest. Space for the light-bodied 'wash' is created by either removing some material from the original impression or by using a spacer (e.g. polythene sheet) when recording the first impression.

19.3 Silicone rubbers (condensation curing)

Composition   These materials may be supplied as two pastes or as a paste and liquid. Whichever method of dispensation is used the principle of the setting reaction is similar and depends on the cross-linking of hydroxyl-terminated polydimethyl-siloxane chains, brought about by an alkyl silicate cross-linking agent and a tin compound as catalyst. The ingredients required for this reaction to occur are reflected in the composition of a typical paste/liquid material, given in Table 19.3. These materials are very similar to the room temperature polymerizing silicones used as denture soft liners (p. 97). Fig. 14.3 gives the structural formula of the silicone prepolymer. The viscosity of the paste is controlled by the amount of inert filler, as in the case of the polysulphides. Light-bodied, regular-

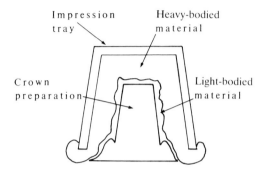

Fig. 19.3 Line diagram showing section of an impression in which heavy-bodied and light-bodied materials have been used to obtain optimal accuracy and dimensional stability.

bodied, heavy-bodied and 'putty' materials are available. The latter is a paste of very high viscosity and its availability denotes an important difference between the silicones and polysulphides.

Proportioning of the paste/liquid materials is by mixing a given volume of paste with a fixed number of drops of liquid. For paste/paste materials equal lengths of pastes are mixed together. A colour contrast between the pastes enables the operator to see when proper mixing has been achieved.

Setting reaction   On mixing the two components, either two pastes or paste and liquid, a reaction begins immediately in which the terminal hydroxyl groups of prepolymer chains react with the cross-linking agent under the influence of the catalyst (Fig. 14.3). Each molecule of cross-linking agent may, potentially, react with up to four prepolymer chains causing extensive cross-linking. Each reaction stage also produces one molecule of ethyl alcohol as a byproduct. Cross-linking produces an increase in viscosity and the rapid development of elastic properties.

Properties   The setting characteristics of the silicone materials tend to be more favourable than those of the polysulphides. Setting times are gen-

Table 19.3 Composition of a paste–liquid silicone rubber impression material (condensation curing)

	Component	Function
Paste	Hydroxyl-terminated polydimethyl-siloxane (liquid, silicone, prepolymer)	Undergoes cross-linking to form rubber.
	Insert filler such as silica	Gives 'body', controls viscosity and modifies physical properties.
Liquid	Alkyl silicate such as tetra-ethylsilicate	Acts as cross-linking agent.
	Tin compound such as dibutyl tin dilaurate	Acts as reaction catalyst.

erally shorter and elasticity is developed earlier.

The set material has adequate tear resistance for most purposes. A regular-bodied silicone material can undergo only about 300 percent extension before fracturing, (compared to 700 percent for polysulphides) but most of this strain is recoverable. The silicones have elastic properties which most closely approach the ideal of complete and instantaneous recovery following stretching or compression.

Many of the properties are related to the filler content of the pastes. The trends are identical to those given in Table 19.2 for polysulphides. In the case of the silicones an additional, very high viscosity or 'putty' paste exists which has even lower setting and thermal contraction values than the conventional heavy-bodied materials. It also has better dimensional stability.

Dimensional changes after setting, for condensation curing silicones, may be due to continued slow setting or due to loss of alcohol produced as a byproduct of the setting reaction. The latter effect produces a measurable weight loss which is accompanied by a shrinkage of the impression material. Dimensional changes of regular-bodied condensation silicones are slightly greater than those of regular-bodied polysulphides but are small compared to the changes which occur with alginates. In order to obtain optimum accuracy, the models should be cast as soon as possible after recording the impression.

Silicone elastomers may be considered essentially non-toxic, despite the fact that they contain a heavy metal catalyst. The materials are extremely hydrophobic and are in the patient's mouth for only a few minutes. The liquid component of the paste/liquid materials may be hazardous if not handled carefully. Accidental splashes may cause considerable irritation and blistering of the eyes.

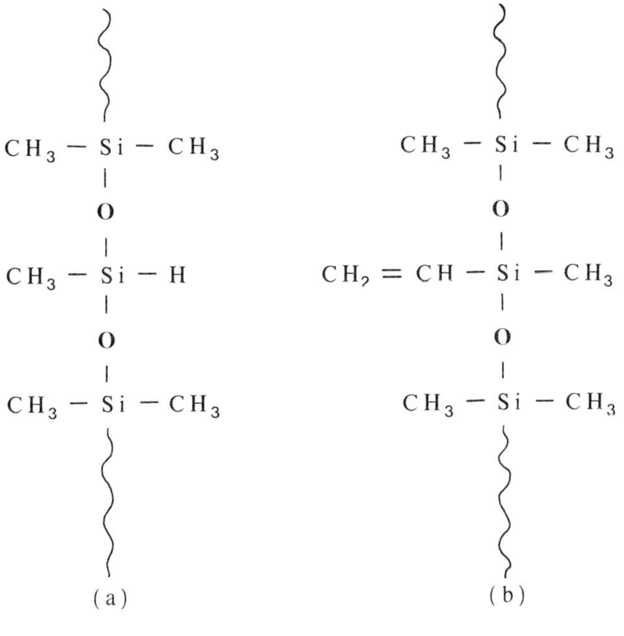

Fig. 19.4 Structural formulae of the silicone prepolymers used in the two pastes of addition curing silicone impression materials. (a) One paste contains some Si–H groups. (b) The other paste contains some Si–CH=CH$_2$ groups.

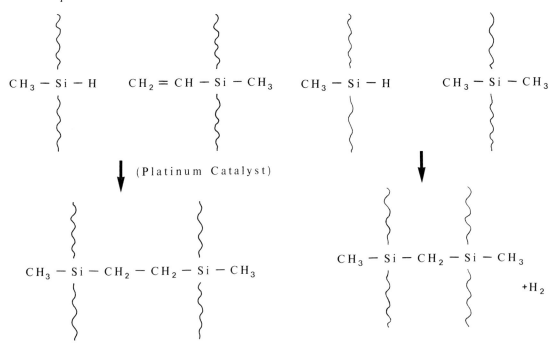

Fig. 19.5 Platinum-catalysed addition reaction which causes cross-linking of prepolymer chains.

Fig. 19.6 Schematic representation of a possible mechanism by which hydrogen can be produced with addition curing silicones. This may be responsible for the surface porosity *occasionally* seen on casts.

Applications Condensation silicone rubbers are commonly used for crown and bridge and occasionally for partial denture patients. They are most widely used with stock trays, offering an advantage over the polysulphides which are used almost exclusively with special trays. The advantage accures from the availability of the putty material with its increased accuracy and stability. This is used in combination with a light-bodied material using techniques akin to those described for polysulphides in the previous section.

19.4 Silicone rubbers (addition curing)

Composition These materials are supplied as two pastes. Each paste contains a liquid silicone prepolymer and filler and one of the pastes contains a catalyst. One paste contains a polydimethylsiloxane prepolymer in which some of the methyl groups are replaced by hydrogen (Fig. 19.4a). The other paste contains a prepolymer in which some methyl groups are replaced by vinyl groups (Fig. 19.4b). One of the pastes contains a catalyst which is

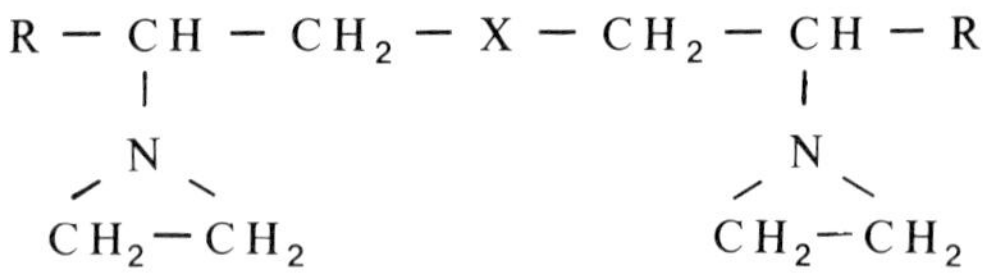

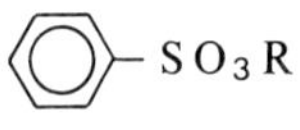

Fig. 19.7 (a) Simplified structural formula of the imine-terminated ether prepolymer present in the base paste of a polyether impression material. X represents repeating units of ethers. (b) Structural formula of an aromatic sulphonic acid ester. This is the main active ingredient of the catalyst paste of a polyether impression material. Group R is an alkyl group, for example, butyl.

normally a platinum-containing compound such as chloroplatinic acid. Four viscosities are available depending on the amount of filler incorporated by the manufacturer.

Proportioning is carried out by extruding equal lengths of each paste onto the mixing pad. A good colour contrast between the pastes enables thorough mixing to be achieved.

Setting reaction On mixing the two pastes a platinum-catalysed addition reaction occurs, causing cross-linking between the two types of siloxane prepolymer (Fig. 19.5). It is noteworthy that the reaction does not involve the production of byproducts although it has been reported that these materials occasionally evolve hydrogen. This is possibly produced by a reaction such as that shown in

Table 19.4 Composition of polyether impression materials

Component		Function
Base paste (large tube)	Imine terminated prepolymer.	Becomes cross-linked to form rubber.
	Inert filler.	To give 'body', control viscosity and physical properties.
Catalyst paste (small tube)	Ester derivative of aromatic sulphonic acid.	Initiates cross-linking.
	Inert oils)	To form paste.
	Inert fillers)	

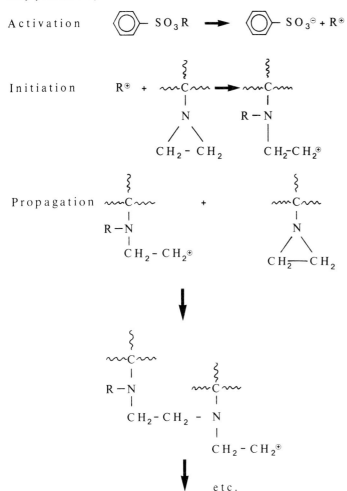

Fig. 19.8 Schematic representation of the cationic, ring opening polymerization involved in the setting of polyether impression materials.

Fig. 19.6. Cross-linking produces an increase in viscosity coupled with the development of elastic properties.

Properties In most respects, the addition curing silicone rubbers have properties similar to those of the condensation type. They have adequate setting characteristics and tear resistance coupled with near ideal elasticity. The combined use of putty and light-bodied materials enables accurate impressions to be recorded. The most significant difference between the addition curing and condensation curing materials is in their relative dimensional stability. The production of little or no byproduct in the cross-linking reaction of the addition curing material results in a very stable impression.

Applications These materials are used primarily for crown and bridge and occasionally for partial denture work. They offer a significant advantage in cases where models cannot be cast soon after recording the impression since they are known to remain dimensionally stable over a considerable period of time. Stock trays are generally used in techniques employing both putty and light-bodied pastes. A special tray may be required if a heavy-bodied/light-bodied combination is used.

19.5 Polyethers

Composition These materials are normally supplied as two pastes. The 'base' paste, containing the prepolymer and inert filler is supplied in a large tube. The 'catalyst' paste, containing a reaction initiator together with paste-forming oils and fillers, is supplied in a second, but much smaller tube. The composition is summarized in Table 19.4. Simplified structural formulae for the imine-terminated, ether prepolymer and the aromatic sulphonic acid ester initiator are given in Fig. 19.7. The materials are generally supplied in only one viscosity, equivalent to the regular-bodied materials of other elastomers. The manufacturers do supply a diluent oil, however, which can be used to produce a paste with viscosity akin to that of a light-bodied material.

The two pastes are proportioned by volume. Equal lengths of paste are extruded onto a mixing pad giving a base paste/catalyst paste volume ratio of about 8:1. The good colour contrast between the pastes aids mixing.

Setting reaction When the two pastes are mixed together a cationic, ring opening addition polymerization occurs. The ionized form of the sulphonic acid ester provides the initial source of cations and each stage of the reaction involves the opening of an epimine ring and the production of a fresh cation, as illustrated in Fig. 19.8. Distinct activation, initiation and propagation stages may be identified in the reaction as shown. The reaction is of the addition type with no byproduct being produced. Since each prepolymer molecule has two reactive epimine groups, individual propagation

Table 19.5 Comparison of the properties of elastomeric impression materials

Property	Polysulphides	Condensation silicones	Addition silicones	Polyethers
Viscosity	Available in 3 viscosities (no putty)	Available in 4 viscosities including putty	Available in 4 viscosities including putty	Available in a single viscosity (regular) + diluent
Tear resistance	Good	Adequate	Adequate	Adequate
Elasticity	Viscoelastic material	Very good	Very good	Adequate
Accuracy	Good with special trays	Acceptable with stock trays	Good with stock trays	Good with special trays
Dimensional stability	Adequate, but pouring of models should not be delayed*	Models should be poured as quickly as possible*	Very good*	Very good in low humidity conditions

*Some manufacturers recommend a *short* delay in pouring models for these materials, either to allow elastic recovery to occur or to allow gaseous products to escape which would otherwise cause pitting of the model surface.

reactions may produce simple chain lengthening or cross-linking. As the reaction proceeds, the viscosity increases and eventually a relatively rigid cross-linked rubber is produced.

Properties   The polyether materials have adequate tear resistance and elastic properties approaching those of the silicones. They are relatively rigid when set and considerable force may be required to remove the impression after setting, particularly when the undercuts are severe.

The accuracy of polyether impressions compares favourably with other regular-bodied elastomers. The lack of heavy-bodied and putty pastes, however, precludes the use of techniques using combined viscous/fluid pastes which are commonly used with other elastomers to optimize accuracy.

Under conditions of low relative humidity, the polyether materials have very good dimensional stability. This is related, primarily, to the fact that the material contains no volatile constituents and sets by an addition reaction which produces no volatile byproducts. The set material is relatively hydrophilic and absorbs water under conditions of high humidity. This causes the impression material to swell and distort. The use of polyether materials should therefore be avoided in climates where humidity is high and where efficient air conditioning is not available.

Applications   Polyethers are commonly used in crown and bridge work and occasionally for other applications. The materials are said to be suitable for use with either stock trays or special trays. The latter are preferable, however, in view of the lack of high-viscosity, heavy-bodied or putty pastes.

19.6 Comparison of the properties of elastomers

Table 19.5 gives an indication of the comparative properties of the four types of elastomeric impression material. The final choice of material is often a matter of personal preference on the part of the clinician.

20

Requirements of Direct Filling Materials

20.1 Introduction

Direct filling materials are used for chairside restoration of teeth. They differ from indirect restorations, such as crowns, bridges or inlays, because no laboratory stage is involved in the provision of the restoration.

Teeth may need restoring for a variety of reasons. Destruction of tooth substance caused by dental caries may result in the loss of considerable quantities of enamel and dentine. Trauma may cause fracture and loss of parts of teeth. In this case the anterior teeth are most vulnerable and those teeth affected may be otherwise sound and caries-free. A third factor causing loss of tooth substance is abrasion. This often arises due to overzealous brushing using an abrasive dentrifice but may also arise due to a peculiarity of the diet, working environment or habits of the patient.

The parts of teeth which require replacement by a restorative material vary in size, shape and location in the mouth. Thus, at one extreme, it may be necessary to restore a large cavity which extends over the mesial, occlusal and distal surfaces of a molar tooth. An entirely different situation is the restoration of the corner of an incisor which has been lost in an accident. The requirements of materials used in these and other applications vary and it is not surprising that no single restorative material is suitable for all cases. For some situations the strength and abrasion resistance of the material may be the prime consideration. In other situations appearance and adhesive properties may become more important.

The factor which is generally used to assess the success or failure of a restorative material for any application is *durability*. In this context the term refers to the life expectancy of the restoration and the life expectancy of the surrounding tooth substance and how it may be affected by the presence of the restoration. Durability depends on the physical and biological properties of the restorative material.

The acceptance of the material by the profession also depends on the ease with which it can be handled in the surgery.

20.2 Rheological properties and setting characteristics

Many restorative materials are supplied as two or more components which require mixing. Thorough mixing should be easy to accomplish in a reasonable time. After mixing, the ease of handling depends on factors such as *viscosity*, 'tackiness' and setting characteristics such as *working time* and *setting time*. Different techniques must often be adopted to handle different materials. Whereas some materials readily flow into the prepared cavity under little pressure some products require 'packing' under considerable pressure. When materials remain tacky for some time after mixing they may be difficult to handle because they adhere to instruments. Working time should be sufficiently long to enable manipulation and placement of materials before the setting reaction reaches the stage where continued manipulation is either difficult or would adversely affect the structure and properties of the final set material. Setting times should, ideally, be short for the comfort and convenience of both the patient and clinician.

20.3 Chemical properties

Filling materials are required to withstand the hostile environment of the oral cavity for many years without dissolving, degrading or eroding. Thus, the materials must withstand large variations in pH and a variety of solvents which may be taken into the mouth in drinks, foodstuffs and medicaments. In addition, metallic filling materials should not undergo excessive corrosion or be involved in the development of electrical currents which may cause *galvanic pain*.

20.4 **Thermal properties**

Filling materials should, ideally, be good thermal insulators, protecting the dental pulp from the harmful effects of hot and cold stimuli. The thermal insulating properties of filling materials are best characterized in terms of *thermal diffusivity* (p. 19) since this describes the behaviour of materials subjected to transient thermal stimuli. Hence, the value of thermal diffusivity should ideally be low. Materials having relatively high values of thermal diffusivity require the use of an insulating cavity base material.

The thermal expansion and contraction of a filling which occurs, for example, when a patient takes a hot or cold drink, should match that of the surrounding tooth substance. Thus, materials should have values of *coefficient of thermal expansion* (p. 21) similar to those of enamel and dentine. A large mismatch of values may result in leakage of fluids down the margin between the filling material and surrounding tooth.

20.5 **Mechanical properties**

The mechanical property requirements of filling materials vary considerably depending on the type of tooth and the particular surface being restored. For the restoration of large cavities, involving two or more surfaces of a posterior tooth, a *strong* material with adequate *abrasion resistance* is required to withstand the large stresses developed in that region of the mouth. When materials are subjected to direct masticatory loading they should also be able to resist plastic deformation or *creep*. For a small occlusal cavity in a posterior tooth the properties of the material may not be as critical since it is totally supported by enamel. For a small interproximal cavity in the anterior region the major factor for consideration may be abrasion resistance. That surface of the tooth is not involved in direct contact with other teeth but may be subjected to considerable toothbrush/dentifrice abuse.

It is recognized that the marginal seal between filling material and tooth substance may be destroyed if the material is able to undergo elastic deformation under loading. A high value of *modulus of elasticity* is therefore beneficial.

20.6 **Adhesion**

It is recognized that an adhesive bond between restorative material and tooth substance is desirable though not always attainable. Such a bond effectively seals the margin, preventing the ingress of fluids and bacteria. In addition, the adhesive bond potentially reduces the amount of cavity preparation required in order to achieve retention of the filling. The subject of adhesion and adhesive materials is dealt with in Chap. 24.

20.7 **Biological properties**

Filling materials, in common with all other dental materials, should be harmless, to both the operators and patients. The specific requirements of these products relate to their effect on the dental pulp. They should not, either directly or indirectly, cause irritation to the pulp, nor should they contain substances which are able to leach out and cause irritation. It should be remembered that dentine contains many tubules which are capable of transporting chemicals from the base of fillings to the pulp. Biologically bland cavity bases or cavity linings are often used when filling materials are not sufficiently bland to be used directly.

Dental Amalgam

21.1 Introduction

An amalgam consists of a mixture of two or more metals, one of which is mercury. Dental amalgam consists, essentially, of mercury combined with a powdered silver–tin alloy. Mercury is a liquid at room temperature and is able to form a 'workable' mass when mixed with the alloy. This behaviour renders the material suitable for use in dentistry.

The reaction between mercury and alloy which follows mixing is termed an *amalgamation* reaction. It results in the formation of a hard restorative material of silvery-grey appearance. The colour generally limits its use to those cavities where appearance is not of primary concern.

Dental amalgam has been used for many years with a large measure of success, in fact, it is the most widely used of all the available filling materials.

21.2 Composition

Mercury used in dental amalgam is purified by distillation. This ensures the elimination of impurities which would adversely affect the setting characteristics and physical properties of the set amalgam.

The composition of the alloy powder particles varies from one product to another. Many alloys, conveniently described as *conventional alloys*, have a composition in which the concentrations of the component metals are as given in Table 21.1. It can be seen that the major components of the alloy are silver, tin and copper. Small quantities of zinc and mercury are also present in some alloys. The composition limits given in Table 21.1 formed the basis of many national standard specifications for amalgam alloy for many years.

The quantities of silver and tin specified ensure a preponderance of the silver/tin intermetallic compound Ag_3Sn. This compound, known as the γ (gamma) phase of the silver–tin system, is formed

Table 21.1 Composition of 'conventional' amalgam alloys

Metal	Weight percentage
Silver	65 (minimum)
Tin	29 (maximum)
Copper	6 (maximum)
Zinc	2 (maximum)
Mercury	3 (maximum)

over only a small composition range and is particularly advantageous since it readily undergoes an amalgamation reaction with mercury. Most conventional alloys contain around 5 percent copper, which has a significant strengthening effect on the set amalgam.

The role of zinc is as a *scavenger* during the production of the alloy. The alloy is formed by melting all the constituent metals together. At the elevated temperatures required for this purpose there is a tendency for oxidation to occur. Oxidation of tin, copper or silver would seriously affect the properties of the alloy and amalgam. Zinc reacts rapidly and preferentially with the available oxygen, forming a slag of zinc oxide which is easily removed. Many alloys contain no zinc. They are described as *zinc-free alloys* and oxidation during melting is prevented by carrying out the procedure in an inert atmosphere.

The majority of alloy powders contain no mercury. Those products containing up to 3 percent mercury are called *pre-amalgamated alloys*. They are said to react more rapidly when mixed with mercury.

The shape and size of the alloy powder particles vary from one product to another. Two methods are commonly used to produce the particles. Firstly, filings of alloy may be cut from a prehomogenized ingot of alloy. These *lathe-cut* alloy powders are irregular in shape (Fig. 21.1a) and are graded according to size, being described as fine-

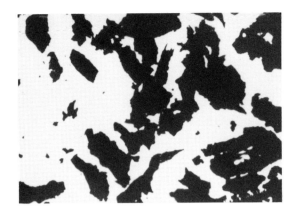

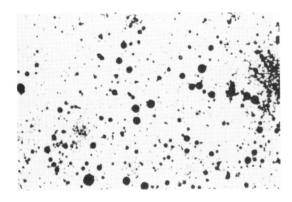

Fig. 21.1 Dental amalgam alloys. (a) Lathe-cut alloy particles (× 70). (b) Spherical alloy particles (× 70).

grain or coarse-grain. Secondly, particles may be produced by *atomization*. Here, molten alloy is sprayed into a column filled with inert gas. The droplets of alloy solidify as they fall down the column. Particles produced in this way are either *spherical* or *spheroidal* in nature (Fig. 21.1b).

Many alloy powders are formulated by mixing particles of varying size or even shape in order to increase the packing efficiency of the alloy and reduce the amount of mercury required to produce a workable mix.

Many alloys produced over recent years cannot be described as 'conventional' since they have a composition markedly different from that given in Table 21.1. Although they have the same basic ingredients, they contain much more copper, typically between 10 and 30 percent, compared to less than 6 percent in the conventional alloys. These newer alloys are referred to as *copper-enriched alloys*. In addition to the increased copper levels some alloys also contain small quantities of

other metals such as palladium. Higher copper levels in alloy powders may be produced by the manufacturer in one of several ways. Lathe-cut. spherical or spheroidal powders can be produced in which the manufacturer alters the ratio of metals at the melting stage. Hence the resulting alloy particles are similar in shape and size to conventional alloys but simply contain a higher copper content. These are *single-composition, copper-enriched alloys*. An alternative approach is to blend particles of conventional alloy with those of, for example, a silver–copper alloy in order to achieve a higher overall copper content. Such blends are called *dispersion-modified, copper-enriched alloys* and one widely used product contains two parts by weight of a lathe-cut alloy of conventional composition (less than 6 percent copper) and one part by weight of spherical silver–copper eutectic particles (Fig. 21.2). The latter particles contain 72 parts silver and 28 parts copper and the overall copper content in the blended alloy is 12 percent.

21.3 Setting reactions

The reaction which takes place when alloy powder and mercury are mixed is complex. Mercury diffuses into the alloy particles; very small particles may become totally dissolved in mercury. The alloy structure of the surface layers is broken down and the constituent metals undergo amalgamation with mercury. The reaction products crystallize to give new phases in the set amalgam. A considerable quantity of the initial alloy remains unreacted at the completion of setting. The structure of the set material is such that the unreacted cores of alloy particles remain embedded in a matrix of reaction products.

In simplified terms, the reaction for conventional amalgam alloys may be given by the following unbalanced equation.

$$Ag_3Sn + Hg \rightarrow Ag_2Hg_3 + Sn_xHg + Ag_3Sn$$
$$\text{or} \quad \gamma + Hg \rightarrow \gamma_1 + \gamma_2 + \gamma$$

The primary reaction products are a silver–mercury phase (the γ_1 phase) and a tin–mercury phase (the γ_2 phase). The γ_2 phase has a rather imprecise structure and the value of x in the formula Sn_xHg may vary from 7 to 8. The equation emphasizes the fact that considerable quantities of unreacted alloy (γ phase) remain unconsumed.

For copper-enriched alloys the reaction may be represented by:

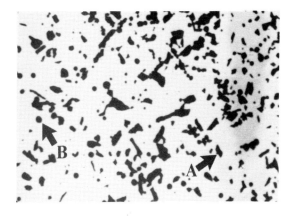

Fig. 21.2 Dispersion-modified alloy powder. Lathe-cut particles of conventional alloy (A) and spherical particles of silver—copper eutectic alloy (B). (× 70)

$$Ag_3Sn + Cu + Hg \rightarrow Ag_2Hg_3 + Cu_6Sn_5 + Ag_3Sn$$
$$\text{or } \gamma + Cu + Hg \rightarrow \gamma_1 + Cu_6Sn_5 + \gamma$$

The essential difference between this and the reaction for conventional alloys is the replacement of the tin—mercury, γ_2 phase in the reaction product with a copper—tin phase.

In the case of the dispersion-modified, copper-enriched materials, it is believed that the particles of conventional lathe-cut alloy initially react to form γ_1 and γ_2 phases. The γ_2 phase then reacts with copper from the silver—copper eutectic spheres to form the copper—tin phase. Thus, in these materials, the γ_2 phase exists as an intermediate reaction product for a short time during setting.

The reaction rate is quite slow and sometimes takes several days or even weeks to reach completion. This is reflected in the rate of development of mechanical properties.

21.4 Properties

Dimensional changes The setting reaction for amalgam involves a dimensional change. If cylindrical specimens of material are prepared and allowed to set in unrestrained conditions, plots of dimensional change versus time are akin to those shown in Fig. 21.3. Curves (a) and (b) are typical of results obtained for commonly used materials. A small contraction takes place during the first half hour or so. This corresponds to the stage during which mercury is still diffusing into the alloy particles. The upturn in the curve begins when crystallization

of new phases becomes the predominant feature of the setting reaction. The outward thrust of growing crystals causes the expansion. The overall effect may cause a slight final expansion as shown in curve (a) or a slight final contraction as in curve (b). Factors which affect the amount of expansion or contraction include the type of alloy used, the particle size and shape and, most significantly, manipulative variables such as the pressure used to condense the amalgam into the cavity. It is important that the final set filling should not have dimensions which are very different from that of the cavity. A large contraction would result in a marginal gap down which fluids could penetrate. A large expansion would result in the protrusion of the filling from the cavity. Hence, standard specification tests for dental amalgam permit only a small expansion (typically 0·2 percent maximum) or a small contraction (typically 0·1 percent maximum).

A far greater expansion may result if a zinc-containing amalgam is contaminated with moisture during condensation. Zinc reacts readily with water producing hydrogen.

$$Zn + H_2O \rightarrow ZnO + H_2$$

The liberation of hydrogen causes a considerable *delayed expansion* as illustrated by curve (c) in Fig. 21.3. This confirms the need for adequate moisture control when using these materials.

Strength The strength of dental amalgam is developed slowly. It may take up to 24 hours to reach a reasonably high value and continues to increase slightly for some time after that. At the time when the patient is dismissed from the surgery, typically some 15—20 minutes after placing the filling, the amalgam is relatively weak. It is necessary, therefore, to instruct patients not to apply undue stress to their freshly placed amalgam fillings.

Spherical particle alloys and copper-enriched alloys develop strength more rapidly than conventional lathe-cut materials. Fine-grain, lathe-cut products develop strength more rapidly than coarse-grain products (Fig. 21.4). There is little difference in the ultimate compressive strength values of the materials — all being adequate in this respect.

The tensile strength and transverse strength values of amalgam are very much lower than the compressive strength. The material is weak in thin sections and unsupported edges of amalgam are readily fractured under occlusal loads. Due regard must be paid to the mechanical properties of amalgam when considering cavity preparation. The

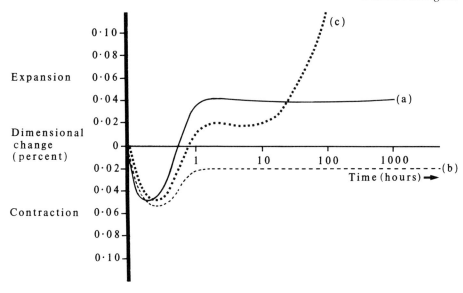

Fig. 21.3 Dimensional change versus time for dental amalgam. Measurements started soon after mixing. (a) and (b) Examples of normal behaviour. (c) Example of moisture-contaminated material.

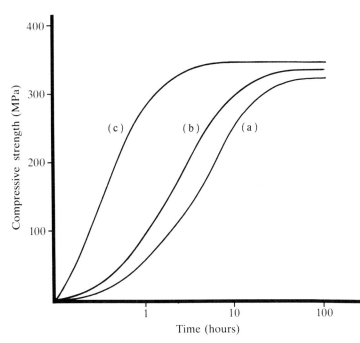

Fig. 21.4 Graph showing increase in compressive strength as a function of time. (a) Coarse-grain, lathe-cut material. (b) Fine-grain, lathe-cut material. (c) Spherical particle material.

material should be considered essentially brittle in nature, requiring adequate support from surrounding structures and occasionally requiring reinforcement with metal pins embedded in dentine. Technique may play an important part in determining the final strength of amalgam. There is good correlation between strength and mercury content. Optimum properties are produced for amalgams containing 44–48 percent mercury. Since most materials are initially proportioned at more than 50 percent mercury it is necessary to reduce this level during manipulation.

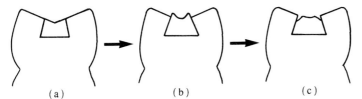

Fig. 21.5 Diagram showing how creep of amalgam causes the formation of unsupported edges which can fracture. (a) Initial restoration. (b) Following creep. (c) Following marginal fracture.

Plastic deformation (creep)   Amalgam undergoes a certain amount of plastic deformation or creep when subjected to dynamic intra-oral stresses. The tendency for a material to creep is, however, normally measured in the laboratory using a *static creep* test. (See p. 16.)

The significance of creep can be explained by reference to Fig. 21.5. Creep causes the amalgam to flow, such that unsupported amalgam protrudes from the margin of the cavity (Fig. 21.5b). These unsupported edges are weak and may be further weakened by corrosion. Fracture causes the formation of a 'ditch' around the margins of the amalgam restoration. The phenomenon is often referred to as the *ditching* of amalgam. The γ_2 phase of amalgam is primarily responsible for the relatively high values of creep exhibited by some materials. The copper-enriched amalgams, which contain little or no γ_2 in the set material, have significantly lower creep values and clinical trials show they are less prone to ditching. Amalgams produced from copper-enriched alloys containing small quantities of metals such as palladium or indium have lower values still. This suggests that although the γ_2 phase may be implicated as being responsible for high creep it is not the only factor involved. Typical values of static creep for three types of amalgam are given in Table 21.2.

Corrosion   The term corrosion should be distinguished from the often misused term tarnish. Tarnishing simply involves the loss of lustre from the surface of a metal or alloy due to the formation of a surface coating. The integrity of the alloy is not affected and no change in mechanical properties would be expected. Amalgam readily tarnishes due to the formation of a sulphide layer on the surface.

Corrosion is a more serious matter which may significantly affect the structure and mechanical properties.

The heterogeneous, multiphase structure of dental amalgam makes it prone to corrosion. Electrolytic cells are readily set up in which different phases form the anode and cathode and saliva provides the electrolytes (p. 25).

The γ_2 phase of a conventional amalgam is the most electrochemically reactive and readily forms the anode in an electrolytic cell. The γ_2 phase breaks down to give tin-containing corrosion products and mercury which is able to combine with unreacted alloy (γ phase). The rate of corrosion is accelerated if the amalgam filling contacts a gold restoration. The large difference in potential results in a significant corrosion current being established.

Corrosion produces a restoration with poor appearance and may significantly affect mechanical properties. The chances of ditching are increased, particularly if creep has also occurred. One beneficial effect of corrosion is thought to be the sealing of the margins of the filling with corrosion products which reduces marginal leakage. The level of corrosion can be minimized by polishing the surfaces of restorations. Smooth surfaces are less prone to concentration cell corrosion.

Copper-enriched amalgams contain little or no γ_2 phase. The copper–tin phase, which replaces γ_2 in these materials, is still the most corrosion-prone phase in the amalgam. The corrosion currents produced, however, are orders of magnitude lower than those for conventional amalgams.

It is now generally accepted that copper-enriched amalgams perform better than conventional materials in terms of corrosion and that this may be a factor involved in the lower incidence of ditching reported for these materials. There are no reports of increased marginal leakage for the copper-

Table 21.2 Values of static creep for amalgam

Material type	Creep percentage*
Conventional lathe-cut	3·5
Dispersion-modified, copper-enriched	0·2
Copper-enriched, containing 0·5 percent palladium	0·06

* Creep after 7 days, stress of 37 MPa applied for 4 hours.

enriched materials, indicating that sufficient quantities of corrosion product are produced to seal the margins.

Thermal properties Amalgam has a relatively high value of *thermal diffusivity*, as would be expected for a metallic restorative material. Thus, in constructing an amalgam restoration, an insulating material, dentine, is replaced by a good thermal conductor (Table 21.3). In large cavities it is necessary to line the base of the cavity with an insulating, cavity lining material prior to condensing the amalgam. This reduces the harmful effects of thermal stimuli on the pulp.

The *coefficient of thermal expansion* value for amalgam is about three times greater than that for dentine (Table 21.3). This, coupled with the greater diffusivity of amalgam, results in considerably more expansion and contraction in the restoration than in the surrounding tooth when a patient takes hot or cold food or drink. Such a mismatch of thermal expansion behaviour may cause microleakage around the filling since there is no adhesion between amalgam and tooth substance. The occurrence of decay in the dentine which surrounds an amalgam filling is the major cause for replacement of such restorations. It is likely that microleakage plays an important part in initiating such lesions.

Biological properties Certain mercury compounds are known to have a harmful effect on the central nervous system. Whilst it is generally agreed that amalgam fillings cause little damage to patients, concern has been expressed over the possible effects of long-term exposure of dentists and assistants to mercury vapour. Mercury vapour may be released into the atmosphere during trituration, condensation or during the removal of old amalgam restorations. In addition, spillages of mercury in the surgery can cause long-term contamination of the atmosphere.

Serious problems can be avoided by ensuring

that the surgery is well ventilated and that flooring of a suitable type is chosen such that accidental spillages can be readily dealt with. Excess, waste or scrap amalgam should be stored, under water or chemical fixative solution, in a sealed container in order to prevent another possible source of contamination.

21.5 Manipulative variables

The manipulation of amalgam involves the following sequence of events:
(1) Proportioning and dispensing,
(2) Trituration,
(3) Condensation,
(4) Carving,
(5) Polishing.

The way in which each of these operations is carried out has an effect on the properties of the final restoration.

Proportioning and dispensing Alloy/mercury ratios vary between 5:8 and 10:8. Those mixes containing greater quantities of mercury are 'wetter' and are generally used with hand mixing. Those mixes containing smaller quantities of mercury are 'drier' and are generally used with mechanical mixing. For any given alloy/mercury ratio, the nature of the mix may vary depending upon the size and shape of the alloy particles. Spherical particle alloys, for example, require less mercury to produce a workable mix.

For optimum properties, the final set amalgam should contain less than 50 percent mercury. Those materials used at alloy/mercury ratios at or approaching 5:8 require the removal of excess mercury following trituration and during condensation.

Various methods of dispensation are available. The most accurate method is to weigh the mercury and alloy components using a balance. This method is rarely used however, and both are commonly proportioned using volume dispensers.

The simplest type of volume dispenser consists of a glass bottle with a plastic, screw-top cap. The cap has a spring-loaded plunger which releases a known volume of either mercury or alloy when depressed. This method of dispensation is relatively accurate and reproducible for mercury but less so for the powdered alloys since the amount of alloy released depends on the way in which the particles are packed together in the container.

An alternative method of dispensation for the

Table 21.3 Thermal properties of amalgam and dentine

	Thermal diffusivity $\times 10^{-3}$ cm^2 s^{-1}	Coefficient of thermal expansion $\times 10^{-6}$/°C
Amalgam	78	25
Dentine	2	8

alloy is preproportioned as a powder in a small sachet or envelope or as a tablet in which the powder particles are compressed together. Mixing involves the use of either the contents of one envelope or one tablet with a given volume of mercury.

Perhaps the most commonly used method of dispensation involves the use of semi-automatic dispensers which also carry out the mixing or trituration. These devices typically have two hoppers. One is filled with alloy, the other with mercury. The alloy/mercury ratio can be set by the operator and the required amount of each component is released into a mixing chamber on the throw of a switch or the press of a button.

Another convenient method of dispensation involves the use of encapsulated materials. Each capsule contains both alloy and mercury in proportions which have been determined by the manufacturer. The two components are initially separated by an impermeable membrane which is readily shattered using a purpose-built capsule press or on starting to vibrate the capsule in a mechanical mixer. Capsules which do not require the use of a press are called self-activating capsules.

Trituration The mixing or trituration of amalgam may be carried out by hand, using a mortar and pestle, or in an electrically powered machine which vibrates a capsule containing the mercury and alloy.

For hand trituration, a glass mortar and pestle with roughened surfaces are normally used. A low alloy/mercury ratio (around 5:8) is often required to produce a workable mix and care must be taken not to use excessive pressure during trituration in order to prevent splintering of alloy particles which may change the character of the mix.

The trituration time may have an effect on the properties of the final set amalgam. Some products require at least 40 seconds trituration in order to achieve full 'wetting' of alloy particles by mercury and optimal properties in the amalgam. Following trituration it is necessary to reduce the mercury content of the mix before condensing. This is normally done by placing the amalgam into a strip of gauze or chamois leather and squeezing to express excess mercury which appears as droplets on the outside.

Trituration by hand is not extensively practised in developed countries nowadays. Mechanical mixing is far more widely used. There are three levels of sophistication which may be employed.

Following proportioning, the mercury and alloy may be placed in a capsule which is vibrated on a purpose-built machine, often referred to as an amalgamator. Alternatively, mechanical mixing in a semi-automatic machine, which also proportions mercury and alloy, is possible. The use of encapsulated, preproportioned materials is probably the most convenient, although also the most expensive option. For all three options, trituration times of 5–20 seconds are normal.

The advantages of mechanical trituration are:
(1) A more uniform and reproducible mix is produced,
(2) A shorter trituration time can be used,
(3) A greater alloy/mercury ratio can be used.
This negates the requirement to express excess mercury before condensing. Encapsulated materials have the extra advantage that they are preproportioned by the manufacturer.

Condensation Following trituration, the material is packed or condensed into the prepared cavity using a flat-ended, steel hand instrument called an amalgam condenser. The amalgam is packed in increments, each increment being equivalent to the volume of material which can be carried in an amalgam 'gun'. This is the device used to transfer the material from the mixing vessel to the prepared cavity. During condensation, a fluid, mercury-rich layer is formed on the surface of each incremental layer. The cavity is overfilled and the mercury-rich layer carved away from the surface. This effectively reduces the mercury content of the filling thus improving its mechanical properties.

The technique chosen for condensation must ensure the following:
(1) Adequate adaptation of the material to all parts of the cavity base and walls,
(2) Good bonding between the incremental layers of amalgam,
(3) Optimal mechanical properties in the set amalgam by minimizing porosity and achieving a final mercury content of 44–48 percent.

There should be a minimal time delay between trituration and condensation. If condensation is commenced too late, the amalgam will have achieved a certain degree of set and adaptation, bonding of increments and final mechanical properties are all adversely affected.

There is good correlation between the quality of an amalgam restoration and the energy expended by the operator who condenses it. Hence, best results are achieved by using a high condensing force at a rapid condensing frequency and continuing to condense until the amalgam feels hard and a mercury-rich layer has been formed at the surface. Lower forces are required to condense spherical particle amalgams than lathe-cut materials. There is a danger of displacing a spherical particle material by using a high force, particularly if an amalgam condenser of small diameter is utilized. Mechanical condensers are available. These apply a forced vibration to the surface of the amalgam.

Carving Soon after condensing the amalgam, the surface layer, which is rich in mercury, is carved away with a sharp instrument. Carving should be carried out when the material has reached a certain degree of set. If attempts are made to carve too soon there is a danger of 'dragging out' significant amounts of material from the surface. If carving is delayed too long the material may become too hard to carve and there is a danger of chipping at the margins.

Spherical amalgams are easier to carve than lathe-cut materials and fine-grain products easier than coarse-grain.

Polishing Polishing is carried out in order to achieve a lustrous surface having a more acceptable appearance and better corrosion resistance. The fillings should not be polished until the material has achieved a certain level of mechanical strength, otherwise there is a danger of fracture, particularly at the margins. The strength which should be attained before polishing is commenced is not certain but many products require a delay of 24 hours between placing and polishing. It is claimed that some faster setting materials can be polished soon after placing. Following initial finishing with multifluted burs, methods used for polishing amalgams include mixtures of pumice in glycerine, zinc oxide in alcohol or ceric oxide in water in combination with a bristle brush or rubber cup in a slow-speed dental handpiece.

22

Silicate Filling Materials (Silicate Cements)

22.1 Introduction

Silicates were the earliest of the 'direct' tooth-coloured filling materials. They have been available since the beginning of the 20th century and have changed little, in terms of composition, since then. The durability of a silicate restoration depends critically on the care taken in handling the material and on the oral hygiene of the patient. Thus, silicate restorations may have a lifetime of only a few months or less or, on the other hand, may last twenty years or more.

22.2 Composition

The materials are normally supplied as a powder and liquid which are mixed together.

The powder is a sodium aluminosilicate glass which is formed by fusing the various glass-making components in the presence of about 20 percent calcium fluoride. The latter compound acts as a flux, aiding the fusion of the glass and ensuring a material of homogeneous composition. The fused glass is pulverized to form a powder, then sieved to give the desired particle size distribution.

The liquid is a buffered, aqueous solution of phosphoric acid of approximately 50 percent concentration. The buffers are normally soluble phosphates such as zinc phosphate or aluminium phosphate. They are added in order to stabilize the pH of the liquid against the effects of small changes in concentration, due to evaporation or condensation of water, and to produce a material with controlled and predictable setting characteristics.

22.3 Setting reaction

The reaction which occurs when powder and liquid are mixed together is fairly complex. In simplified terms it may be regarded as a series of acid−base reactions in which metal ions in the glass react with phosphoric acid to form a series of phosphate salts.

$$Al^{3+} + H_3PO_4 \rightarrow AlPO_4 + 3H^+$$
$$Ca^{2+} + H_3PO_4 \rightarrow CaHPO_4 + 2H^+$$
$$Na^+ + H_3PO_4 \rightarrow NaH_2PO_4 + H^+$$

A more descriptive indication of what occurs is given in Fig. 22.1. Protons from the dissociated acid penetrate the outer layers of the glass particles, displacing cations which combine with phosphate ions to form the matrix. The principal component of the matrix is thought to be aluminium phosphate which exists as an inorganic polymer and binds the set material together. The core of each glass particle remains unreacted whilst the outer layers form a gel which unites the matrix with the unreacted cores.

When cations are displaced from the outer layers of glass particles they are often associated with fluoride ions. Thus, a relatively high fluoride concentration eventually develops in the matrix areas. Fluoride ions are relatively mobile and are able to diffuse through the matrix to the surface of the restoration, where they are leached into saliva or absorbed by surrounding tooth substance.

22.4 Properties

Setting characteristics The setting reaction is rather slow and protracted. Initial hardening occurs within a few minutes but complete setting may not be achieved for several hours. During the early stages of setting the material is very sensitive to moisture contamination which causes a reduction in strength and increase in solubility. In order to achieve optimum durability it is therefore necessary to place the filling material under dry conditions and to protect it from moisture until fully set. This is achieved by coating the surface with a layer of varnish which gives protection for an hour or so. The varnish is a solution of a resin in a volatile solvent such as ether. The solvent evapo-

(a) $\quad H_3\,PO_4 \rightleftharpoons H^+ + H_2\,PO_4^-$

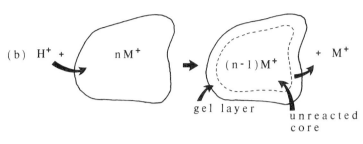

Fig. 22.1 The setting of silicate materials. (a) Formation of protons. (b) Protons enter the outer layers of glass particles, displacing cations. (c) Cations react with phosphate anions to form a matrix of metallic phosphates.

(b) $\quad H^+ +$ nM^+ $(n-1)M^+$ $+ M^+$

gel layer   unreacted core

(c) $\quad M^+ + H_2PO_4^- \longrightarrow MH_2PO_4$

M^+ represents Al^{3+}, Ca^{2+} or Na^+

rates leaving a thin film of resin over the surface.

Drying out After setting, the surface of the material must not be allowed to dry out since it soon dessicates, becomes opaque and cracks. This may be a problem in anterior restorations of mouth-breathing patients for whom the silicate materials cannot be recommended. Drying out may also occur when securing a dry field while operating on an adjacent tooth. Silicate restorations should be coated with varnish before carrying out such procedures.

Appearance The set material has good appearance. A high concentration of unreacted glass cores gives a degree of translucency which, coupled with the availability of a variety of tooth-like shades, enables close matching with surrounding tooth substance. The surface of the restoration is initially smooth and glossy. The high-quality surface finish is impaired if any polishing procedures are carried out and is eventually lost due to a slow process of

erosion. The roughened surface resulting from erosion, with glass particles protruding from the phosphate matrix, may stain to give a further mismatch in appearance between the filling and tooth.

Erosion A major drawback of silicates is their potential to undergo erosion. They erode very slowly at neutral pH but are far less stable if the pH drops much below a value of 5. Plaque pH values are commonly around 4 and, under these conditions, silicates may erode quite rapidly. Restorations produced with a high powder/liquid ratio are less susceptible to erosion than those with a low ratio. This indicates that the matrix phase of the set material is most vulnerable to erosion. Another mechanism of erosion involves the formation of soluble complexes of cement cations with certain anions, particularly citrates. Silicate fillings erode quite rapidly in patients who consume large quantities of fruit juices.

Thermal properties The thermal properties of silicate materials match those of tooth substance more closely than those of most other restorative materials (Table 22.1). Thus, silicates are good thermal insulators and expand and contract at about the same rate as tooth substance.

Fluoride release A significant advantage of silicates is that they slowly release fluoride into surrounding tooth substance, giving a long-term topical fluoride application. The fluoride is able to replace hydroxyl groups in the apatite producing a more acid resis-

Table 22.1 Thermal properties of silicate filling materials compared to tooth substance

	Coefficient of thermal expansion $\times 10^{-6}\ °C$	Thermal diffusivity $\times 10^{-3}\ cm\ s^{-1}$
Silicate material	10	3·4
Enamel	11·4	4·7
Dentine	8·0	2·0

tant structure and it is rare to find secondary caries in the proximity of silicate fillings.

Acidity Due regard must be paid to the acidic nature of silicates at the time of placement. The pH value of freshly mixed cement is around 2·8. The pulp must be protected from the possibly harmful effects of such an acidic material by using a cavity base — normally a calcium hydroxide product. The pH of the cement rises to a value of about 5 after 24 hours.

Mechanical properties Silicates are very brittle materials. They have relatively high values of compressive strength, though not as high as dental amalgam, but very low values of tensile and transverse strength (Table 22.2). They also have low impact strength. The materials are not suitable for use in areas where they may be subjected to high loads or suddenly applied loads. Hence they are not used for class II cavities in posterior teeth or on the biting edges of anterior teeth. They are most widely used for restoring small class III cavities in anterior teeth.

Adhesion Like many other filling materials the silicates show no adhesion to tooth substance. They are retained mechanically by preparing undercut cavities, often at the expense of sound tooth substance.

Table 22.2 Strength of silicate materials compared with amalgam

	Compressive strength MPa	Tensile strength MPa
Silicate	180	15
Amalgam	350	60

22.5 Manipulative variables

Proportioning and mixing It is important to establish a correct powder/liquid ratio for the material being used. The use of too much powder may cause difficulties in mixing and produce a material which is too dry and crumbly to insert into the cavity. The use of excess liquid, on the other hand, produces a fluid mix which has a very low pH value, a long setting time and results in a set material which is very soluble and weak. A powder/liquid ratio of about 4:1 (wt/vol) is about right for hand-mixed materials.

Mixing is carried out on a glass slab. It is advantageous to cool the slab before use. This increases the amount of powder which can be incorporated into a given volume of liquid without giving a dry, crumbly mix. The slab must not be cooled below the dew point temperature however, as this would result in the condensation of water from the

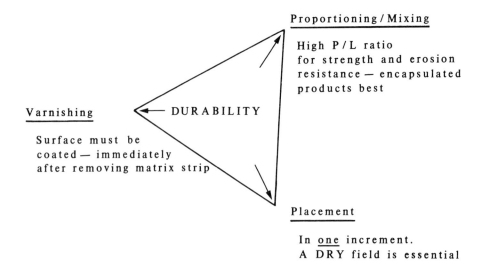

Fig. 22.2 Diagram illustrating the manipulative variables which have an effect on the durability of silicate fillings.

atmosphere. Excess water adversely affects the properties of the material.

Mixing is generally carried out with a stellite or agate spatula. Steel spatulas must not be used since the hard glass particles are capable of abrading steel from the blade. The abraded steel becomes incorporated into the mix, adversely affecting its appearance.

The powder should be incorporated into the liquid in increments and the mixing procedure should be completed quickly in order to ensure sufficient working time. The incorporation of large quantities of powder into the liquid in one go or a prolonged mixing time may reduce the working time to such an extent that the material is difficult to manipulate. A correctly mixed material should have the consistency of putty at the time of insertion into the cavity.

Care must be taken of the liquid component, since there is a tendency for water loss or gain to occur, depending upon the ambient relative humidity. This may adversely affect many properties of the material and is best avoided by ensuring that the liquid container is kept tightly stoppered at all times when not in use.

Encapsulated, mechanically mixed materials have many advantages over hand-mixed products. They are preproportioned by the manufacturer and following only 10 seconds mechanical mixing a putty-like mix is achieved, ready for insertion into the cavity. The powder/liquid ratio is higher than that which can be used for hand-mixed products, producing a stronger, more erosion resistant filling.

Placement of the filling Following mixing, the material is inserted into the prepared and lined cavity in one increment. Incremental packing of silicate materials should be avoided since bonding between layers cannot be guaranteed. It is essential that a dry field is maintained during the placement of the filling, since contamination with moisture at this stage has a drastic effect on the properties of the material. Techniques used to achieve a dry field may vary, depending upon the patient and the location of the tooth. Best results are achieved if the tooth is isolated with a rubber dam.

After placing the material, it is adapted and held under pressure during setting with a plastic *matrix strip*. After setting, the matrix strip is removed and the glossy surface of the set material is immediately covered with a coat of varnish. This protects the material from moisture contamination until setting is well advanced. The surface of the restoration should, ideally, be left undisturbed by the operator. If contouring and polishing cannot be avoided, this process should be delayed for at least 24 hours after placement of the filling.

Fig. 22.2 summarizes the manipulative variables which may have a significant effect on the durability of the filling.

Resin-based Filling Materials

23.1 Introduction

The development of filling materials based on synthetic polymers has been initiated by two major driving forces, in addition to the obvious commercial ones. Firstly, there was a requirement to produce a material which could overcome the major deficiencies of the silicate materials, namely, erosion, brittleness, acidity and a moisture sensitivity which demands very careful manipulation. Secondly, developments in polymer technology produced resins which could be readily cured at mouth temperature and, with the aid of pigments and fillers, could be made to resemble the natural tooth in appearance.

The first materials to be widely used were the *acrylic resins*. These are, essentially, similar to the resins used in denture construction (Chap. 13). The unfilled acrylic resins have now been superceded by a myriad of *composite materials* consisting of a heterogeneous blend of organic resin and inorganic filler.

23.2 Acrylic resins

These are supplied as a powder and liquid which are mixed together. The composition is similar to that given in Table 13.1 for denture base materials.

Table 23.1 Some mechanical properties of acrylic resin, enamel and dentine

	Acrylic resin	Enamel	Dentine
Modulus of elasticity GPa	2	50	15
Compressive strength MPa	70	250	280
Hardness (Vickers)	20	350	60

The pigments used are, generally, white, yellow or brown, in order to match natural tooth shades, as opposed to the pink pigments used in denture base polymers. The setting reaction involves a free radical addition polymerization as described in Chap. 12.

Advantages The acrylic resin materials are *less prone to erosion* than silicates. They have low solubility over a wide range of pH values. They are *less acidic* than silicates though cannot be considered biologically bland due to the presence of residual methylmethacrylate monomer. They are *less brittle* than silicates although their mechanical properties are far from ideal.

The materials are good thermal insulators having a *low value of thermal diffusivity*, $1 \cdot 0 \times 10^{-3} \, \text{cm}^2 \, \text{s}^{-1}$ as opposed to $2 \cdot 0 \times 10^{-3} \, \text{cm}^2 \, \text{s}^{-1}$ for dentine. The ability to match the appearance of tooth substance is, initially, very good, although some products have a tendency to discolour gradually with time. Discolouration at the margins is also observed with many restorations.

Disadvantages Although the acrylic materials do not contain any strong acids, some products contain methacrylic acid, used to modify setting characteristics, and all contain a certain level of residual methylmethacrylate monomer which is *irritant*. This, coupled with a significant *temperature rise* during setting caused by a highly exothermic polymerization reaction, necessitates the use of a protective cavity base material. The material of choice is a setting calcium hydroxide type. Products containing eugenol should be avoided since they retard the setting of the resin and cause discolouration.

The materials undergo a considerable *setting contraction* (6 percent by volume). If uncontrolled, this could produce a significant marginal gap down which fluids could penetrate. The problem may be partially alleviated by filling the cavity with small increments and allowing the contraction to occur

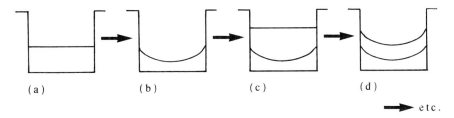

(a)　　　　　(b)　　　　　(c)　　　　　(d)

→ etc.

Fig. 23.1 Diagrammatic representation of incremental layers of acrylic resin filling material, used to partially overcome polymerization contraction. (a) First increment placed. (b) Shrinkage occurs towards base and walls of cavity. (c) Second increment added. (d) Further shrinkage.

towards the walls of the cavity before the next increment is added (Fig. 23.1). Another approach is to overfill the cavity and place the setting material under strong finger pressure with a matrix strip during setting.

The *coefficient of thermal expansion* value for acrylic resin is some 10 times greater than that for tooth substance. The potential for *percolation* of fluids down the restoration–tooth interface when the patient takes hot or cold food and drink is, therefore, significant.

The mechanical properties of acrylic resin compare unfavourably with those of the natural tooth materials which it replaces (Table 23.1). The low value of *modulus of elasticity* indicates that acrylic resin is a far more flexible material than either enamel or dentine. Flexing of restorations under load can lead to marginal breakdown. The lower *compressive strength* and *hardness* values of acrylic resin are reflected in a *poor durability*, particularly when restorations are subjected to abrasive forces. Material loss by *wear* is a phenomenon associated with these relatively soft materials.

Current status Acrylic resins are now rarely used as permanent filling materials. They overcome the major problems associated with silicates but have many other disadvantages which preclude regular use. The materials are still in regular use for temporary crown and bridge construction.

23.3 Composite materials

The addition of reinforcing fillers to resins can have significant effects on properties. The effect depends on the type, shape, size and amount of filler incorporated and, often, the existence of efficient coupling between the filler and resin.

When particulate glass fillers are incorporated in acrylic resins, three properties, namely, coefficient of thermal expansion, setting contraction and surface hardness, depend almost linearly on the filler content, as shown in Fig. 23.2.

Other thermal and mechanical properties may vary in a similar way. Strength and modulus of elasticity generally increase with addition of filler, as does abrasion resistance, probably as a result of increased surface hardness. If the added filler is translucent, the optical properties of the resin are improved and a more lifelike appearance produced.

Classification and composition

Resins All composites consist of a mixture of resin and filler. The nature of the resin may alter slightly from one product to another, although, essentially, they all contain a modified methacrylate or acrylate. Fig. 23.3 gives the molecular structures of two of the most commonly used monomers, Bis GMA and urethane diacrylate, together with that of triethylene glycol dimethacrylate which is a comonomer often used to control the viscosity of the unmixed materials. It can be seen from Fig. 23.3 that the monomer and comonomer molecules are difunctional methacrylates or acrylates. Each carbon–carbon double bond is able to take part in a free radical addition polymerization, to give a highly cross-linked resin after setting.

The size of the monomer and comonomer molecules, coupled with a rapid increase in viscosity during setting, causes a relatively high concentration of acrylate or methacrylate groups to remain unreacted after setting.

Methods of activation Polymerization may be activated *chemically*, by mixing two components, one of which typically contains an initiator and the other an activator, or by an external *ultraviolet* or

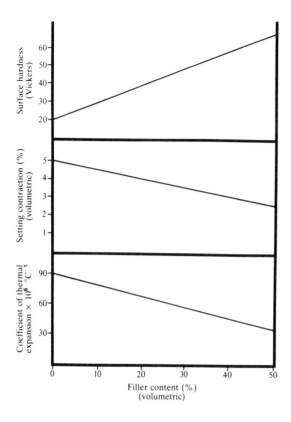

Fig. 23.2 Variation of surface hardness, setting contraction and coefficient of thermal expansion with inorganic filler content for acrylic resins.

visible light source.

For chemical activation, many different methods of dispensation are available. The most popular is the 'two-paste' system. Each paste contains a blend of resin and filler. One paste contains about 1 percent of a peroxide initiator, such as benzoyl peroxide, whilst the other paste contains about 0·5 percent of a tertiary amine activator, such as *N, N′*dimethyl-*p*-toluidine or *p*-tolyl diethanolamine. The ensuing reaction is a free radical addition polymerization as described in Chap. 12.

Other systems which rely on chemical activation are:

(1) Powder/liquid systems, in which the powder contains filler particles and peroxide initiator whilst the liquid contains monomer, comonomer and chemical activator,

(2) Paste/liquid materials in which the paste contains monomers, comonomers, filler and peroxide whilst the liquid contains monomers and chemical activator,

(3) Encapsulated materials in which the filler, mixed with peroxide, is initially separated within a capsule from the monomers and comonomers containing the chemical activator. On breaking the seal between the two parts of the capsule the reactive components come into contact and are mixed mechanically.

Light-activated materials are generally supplied as a single paste which contains monomers, co-monomers, filler and an initiator which is unstable in the presence of either ultraviolet (u.v.) or high-intensity visible light. For u.v.-activated materials, the most commonly used initiator is benzoin methyl ether. At certain selected wavelengths within the u.v. range, this molecule is able to absorb radiation and undergo heterolytic decomposition to form free radicals. The radicals initiate polymerization which then continues in much the same way as that described for vinyl monomers (p. 76).

The use of u.v.-activated materials has diminished greatly since the possible dangers of long-term exposure to ultraviolet radiation were highlighted.

For visible light-activated materials the initiator system comprises a mixture of a diketone and an amine. Camphorquinone is a commonly used diketone which rapidly forms free radicals in the presence of an amine and radiation of the correct wavelength and intensity.

Light-activated materials require the use of a specialist light source, capable of delivering radiation with the appropriate characteristics to the surface of the freshly placed material *in situ*.

Care must be taken in the storage of unused pastes since exposure to sunlight, or particularly to the surgery operating light, may be sufficient to activate a slow initiation process which causes the paste to thicken and become unworkable. For materials which are supplied in pots it is essential to replace the lid quickly after removing the required amount of paste. Many materials are supplied in syringes which will enable the operator or his assistant to expel sufficient material for one restoration. The material remaining in the syringe is not exposed. Another method of dispensation is in the form of 'compules'. Each compule contains sufficient paste for at least one restoration and is extruded into the cavity by placing the compule into a press.

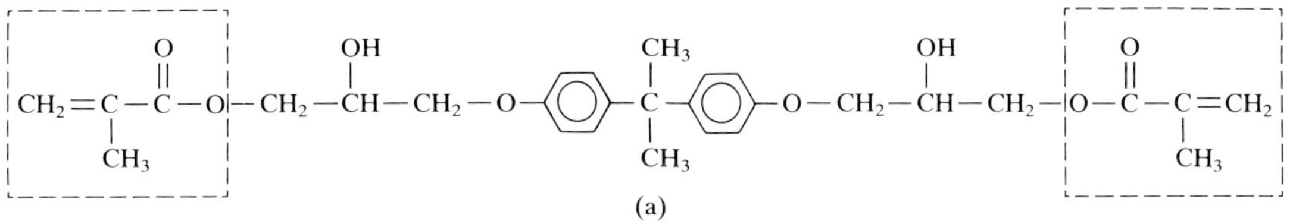

Fig. 23.3 Molecular structures of three modified methacrylate or acrylate resin monomers used in composite materials. (a) Bis GMA (addition product of BisPhenol A and glycidylmethacrylate). (b) Urethane diacrylate. (c) Triethylene glycol dimethacrylate.

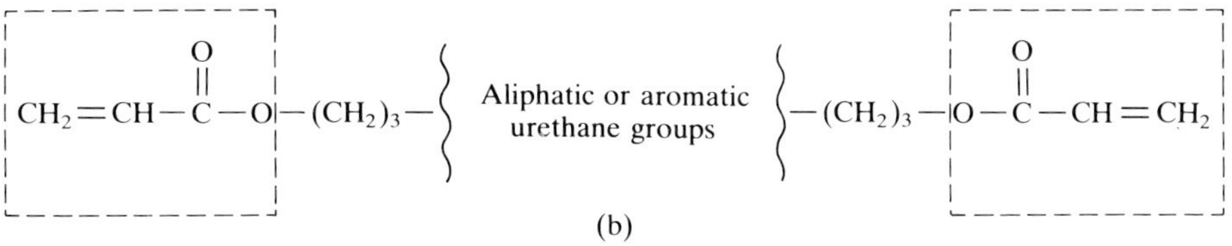

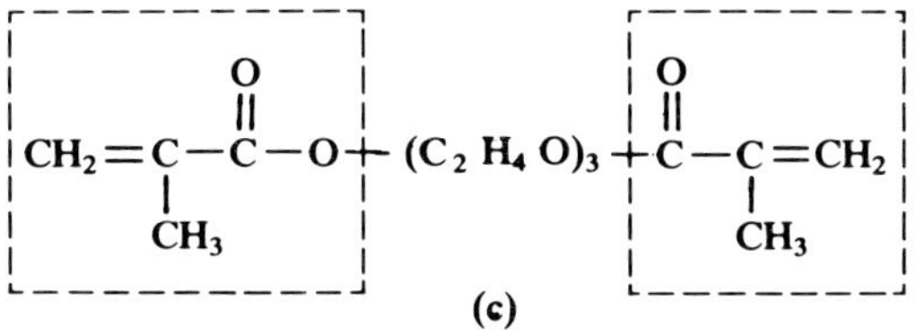

Fillers The type, concentration, particle size and particle size distribution of the filler used in a composite material are major factors controlling properties.

Fillers commonly used include quartz, fused silica and many types of glass including alumino-silicates and borosilicates, some containing barium oxide.

The first generation of composite materials typically contain 60–80 percent, by weight, of quartz or glass in the particle size range of 1–50 μm. The particle size distribution may vary, within this range, from one product to another, some containing relatively greater amounts of larger particles, approaching 50 μm, others containing larger quantities of smaller particles. Materials containing filler particles of this type are normally referred to as *conventional* composites. The filler particles are subjected to a special pretreatment prior to blending with the resin. This involves laying down a surface coating of a *coupling agent* on the particles to enhance bonding between the filler and resin matrix. The coupling agent most commonly used is gamma-methacryloxypropyl-trimethoxysilane.

$$CH_2 = CCH_3CO_2(CH_2)_3Si(OCH_3)_3.$$

This is a difunctional molecule which at one end has the characteristics of a methacrylate monomer whilst at the other it has a silane group capable of interacting and bonding with glass or quartz sur-

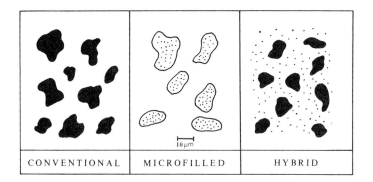

Fig. 23.4 Diagrammatic representation of the size of filler particles used in the three main groups of composite resins.

faces. Hence, it is able to set up a bond between the resin and filler components in a composite system.

Since the composite filling materials were introduced in the mid-1960s, there has been a trend towards the use of fillers with smaller particle size. Many of the currently available products with glass or quartz fillers contain particles in the more limited range of 1–5 μm.

Another development has been the introduction of a number of products containing submicron particles of silica. These materials are referred to as *microfilled composites* and contain silica particles in the range 0·01–0·1 μm with a typical mean diameter of 0·04 μm. The very small particle size produces a massive increase in available surface area for a given volume of filler (typically 10^3–10^4 times more surface area). Subsequently, it is not possible to incorporate very high filler loadings of this small particle size and products which are available contain only 30–60 percent by weight. Even at these lower levels, calculations show that many filler particles must be present as agglomerates and not as individual particles surrounded by resin.

The method of incorporating the smaller particles varies, direct blending with resin being difficult. The most widely used method is to prepare prepolymerized blocks of resin containing a high filler loading of silica. The block is splintered and ground to give particles of resin up to 100 μm in diameter, each containing silica. These particles are blended with monomer, comonomers, initiators or activators to form pastes.

A third series of composite materials contain a blend of both conventional glass or quartz particles together with some submicron, particulate silica.

These products are referred to as *hybrid* composites. Using filler loadings of about 75 percent conventional size (1–50 μm) and 8 percent submicron size (0·40 μm average), a total filler content of 83 percent or greater can be achieved.

Fig. 23.4 shows diagrammatically the microstructure of the three main groups of materials.

Conventional, microfilled and hybrid composites are all available as either chemically activated or light-activated products.

Properties

Setting characteristics For chemically activated materials, setting commences immediately after mixing the two components (paste and paste or paste and liquid etc.). The rate of set is uniform throughout the bulk of the material causing a gradual increase in viscosity at room temperature. Hence, the materials have a limited working time and must be inserted into the prepared cavity before they become unmanageable. After insertion, the materials are held under pressure with a plastic matrix strip and setting is normally completed within two or three minutes. Since setting occurs uniformly throughout the material it is safe to assume that a hard surface indicates that the material has set right through to the base of the cavity. Any material which is not covered by the matrix during setting is likely to have a tacky surface layer due to inhibition of the polymerization reaction by oxygen.

For light-activated materials, only a minimal increase in viscosity takes place before the material is exposed to the activating light source. With these products the operator has, therefore, a longer working time. It should be remembered, however, that visible light-activated materials do begin to set slowly after exposure to light, particularly light of high intensity such as the surgery operating light. Therefore, insertion of the material into the cavity should not be delayed longer than necessary. After being covered with a matrix strip and exposed to the light source, polymerization is often very rapid. Exposure times of between 10 seconds and one minute are, typically, required to cause setting. This ability to set rapidly after exposure to a light source is termed *command setting*.

The pattern of setting for light-activated materials is dictated by the fact that activation is first achieved in the surface layers of material where the light intensity is greatest. The potential for activation declines exponentially as a function of the distance from the surface of the filling. The intensity of light I_x at a distance x from the surface is given by the function:
$$I_x = I_0 \, e^{-\mu x}$$
where I_0 is the light intensity at the surface and μ is the absorption coefficient of the material. Since a certain level of intensity is required to cause activation it follows that light-activated materials have a *limited depth of cure*. The high viscosity of the pastes retards the diffusion of active free radicals from the surface layers to the lower unactivated layers, hence, material which is not activated initially may take a considerable time to set or may remain unset indefinitely.

Manufacturers of light-activated composites can control depth of cure by formulating the products in such a way that they more readily allow light penetration. In addition, they can supply or recommend a light source of adequate intensity and

stipulate the exposure time required to give a certain depth of cure.

Other factors can be controlled by the operator. The distance of the light source from the surface of the material is important. Depth of cure decreases significantly as this distance increases. The operator should never attempt to cure a greater depth of material than that recommended by the manufacturer, nor should he attempt to use a shorter exposure time. When large cavities are being restored the composite material should be cured in increments to ensure proper curing.

Setting contraction The setting contraction of composite resins is considerably smaller than that observed for unfilled acrylic resins. Two factors contribute to this reduction. Firstly, the use of larger monomer and comonomer molecules effectively reduces the concentration of reactive groups in a given volume of material. Secondly, additions of fillers which take no part in the setting reaction further reduce the concentration of reactive methacrylate groups. The setting contraction depends on the number of addition reactions which take place during polymerization and is therefore much smaller for composite materials. Values of around 0·5 percent volumetric contraction are typical as opposed to 6 percent for acrylics.

The contraction, which may be responsible for percolation of fluids at the margins, is offset to some extent by water absorption which causes the material to expand.

Thermal properties The thermal properties of composite materials depend primarily on the filler content. Table 23.2 gives values of thermal diffusivity and coefficient of thermal expansion for a

Table 23.2 Thermal properties of composite resins

	Filler content (percentage by weight)	Thermal diffusivity $\times 10^{-3}$ cm^2 s^{-1}	Coefficient of thermal expansion $\times 10^{-6}$ °C^{-1}
Conventional composite	78	5·0	32
Microfilled composite	50	2·5	60
Unfilled acrylic	0	1·0	90
Dentine	—	2·0	9

conventional composite, microfilled composite, unfilled acrylic resin and dentine for comparison. It can be seen that as the filler content increases the coefficient of thermal expansion decreases, although even for conventional composites, with 78 percent filler, there is still a considerable mismatch in values compared to dentine. This mismatch may cause percolation of fluids down the margins when patients take hot or cold foods. The amount of mismatch which can be tolerated without causing clinically significant problems is not precisely known. It is significant, however, that the microfilled composites have values some 6 or 7 times greater than tooth substance. The thermal diffusivity also depends on filler content although the values for all the materials are close to that measured for dentine and they can all be considered adequate thermal insulators.

Mechanical properties The mechanical properties of composite materials depend upon the *filler content*, the *type of filler*, the efficiency of the filler–resin *coupling* process and the degree of *porosity* in the set material.

Light-activated composites, supplied as single pastes, contain very little porosity whereas chemically activated composites requiring the mixing of two components contain, typically, 2–5 percent porosity. The porosity is introduced during mixing. A correctly cured, light-activated, conventional composite may, typically, have a compressive strength value of 260 MPa, whereas an equivalent chemically activated material, containing 3 percent porosity, is likely to have a compressive strength of 210 MPa. Porosity also has a significant effect on the fatigue limits of composite materials. Nonporous products have a higher fatigue limit and longer fatigue life than porous ones. This may have some bearing on the durability of materials in certain applications.

The lack of an adequate coupling agent pretreatment of the filler may have a dramatic effect on properties. Both the compressive strength and fatigue limit are reduced by about 30 percent when the coupling agent is not used.

Heavily filled, conventional composites undergo brittle fracture. As the filler content is reduced a transition to a more ductile failure is observed. Microfilled composites, which generally have a filler content of 50 percent by weight or less, normally exhibit a yield point at a stress considerably lower than that for fracture. Values of compressive strength for microfilled materials are often similar

Table 23.3 Mechanical properties of composite resins

	Typical conventional composite	Typical microfilled composite	Typical hybrid composite
Compressive strength MPa	260	260	270
Yield stress MPa	260	160	270
Tensile strength MPa	45	40	50
Modulus of elasticity GPa	12	6	14

to or even higher than those for conventional composites, but the lower yield stress value is probably more significant for these products since it represents the point of irretrievable breakdown of the material.

The hybrid composites have mechanical properties very similar to those of conventional materials. Strength and modulus values are often slightly higher but not significantly so. Table 23.3 gives values of certain mechanical properties for typical products from each of the three groups of composite materials. The values of compressive strength are for a porosity-free material.

The significantly lower value of modulus of elasticity for the microfilled materials may have clinical significance. These products may potentially deform under stress, leading to a breakdown of the marginal seal. This is recognized as a problem with unfilled acrylics, where a modulus value of 2 GPa is normal. Whether or not the increase from 2 GPa to 6 GPa is sufficient to prevent breakdown is not known.

Surface characteristics Surface hardness, roughness and abrasion resistance are properties which are mainly controlled by the filler content and particle size.

The resin and filler have characteristic hardness values which remain independent of filler content. The bulk hardness value of the composite, however, increases as the filler content increases. The Vickers hardness number for unfilled resin is about 18 whereas that for a heavily filled conventional composite is about 100. The microfilled materials have values around 40.

The surface of a composite material is initially very smooth and glossy due to contact with a matrix strip during setting. Any process of abrasion, however, has a tendency to cause surface roughening as the relatively soft resin matrix is worn preferentially leaving the filler particles protruding from the surface. This is a particular problem with the conventional and hybrid materials which contain relatively large particles. (Fig. 23.5) One advantage of the microfill materials is that they retain a relatively smooth surface following abrasion, due to the fact that the hard inorganic particles are very small. Another factor which contributes towards surface roughness is the exposure of porosity voids at the surface by abrasion. This is observed for all types of chemically activated composites, and is illustrated in Fig. 23.6 for a microfilled material.

Surface roughness may be caused by abrasive forces exerted on materials during service, for example, from foodstuffs, dentifrices etc. Alternatively, roughening may occur during contouring and polishing. The surface cured against the matrix strip should be left intact if possible, but removal of excess material followed by polishing is often necessary. Table 23.4 gives roughness average values of materials, following polishing by one of three commonly used methods. Values for the smooth, matrix surface are given for comparison.

It can be seen that all of the polishing procedures produce a significant increase in roughness compared to the matrix surface. This is accompanied by a loss of gloss. The increase is greatest for the conventional and hybrid materials and the polishing method which appears most damaging is the use of silicone rubber points.

A smooth surface can be restored to a roughened composite by using a *glazing agent*. These consist of resins which are identical to composites except that they do not contain filler particles. The glaze is applied to the surface of the composite and sets to form a smooth surface layer of about 100 μm thickness. The material is very soft, however, and is soon abraded, revealing the composite surface again.

If the rate of material loss due to abrasion becomes excessive it may cause a change in the anatomical form of the restoration. Abrasion of this magnitude may, conceivably, be caused by one of a variety of mechanisms and is of particular importance when considering the use of composites in posterior cavities. Here, the forces exerted on materials are relatively high and abrasive wear may take place at a rapid pace due to either two-body contacts, normally involving the restorative material and an opposing tooth cusp, or three-body contacts in which an abrasive foodstuff may be involved as the third body between the material and opposing tooth cusp. Cyclic masticatory loadings also offer a potential for fatigue wear in which surface failure occurs following the development of small surface or subsurface cracks over a period of time.

Appearance Composite materials, when freshly placed, offer an excellent match with surrounding tooth substance. The availability of a variety of shades, combined with a degree of translucency imparted by the filler, enables the dentist to achieve a very pleasing result. Polishing reduces the gloss, however, and abrasion may further increase surface roughness. The surface may eventually become stained due to deposition of coloured foodstuffs or

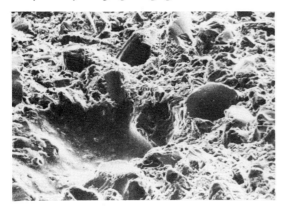

Fig. 23.5 Scanning electron microscope photograph of the roughened surface of a conventional composite material showing protruding filler particles. ($\times$ 750)

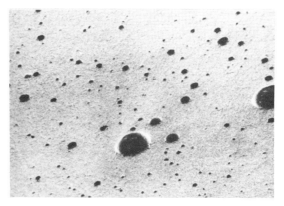

Fig. 23.6 Scanning electron microscope photograph of the abraded surface of a microfilled composite material showing exposed porosity. ($\times$ 325)

Table 23.4 Roughness average (Ra μm) values of composite materials following polishing

Surface treatment	Conventional composite	Microfilled composite	Hybrid composite
None (matrix surface)	0·04	0·02	0·03
Aluminium oxide-impregnated finishing disc	0·15	0·10	0·20
White stone	0·30	0·20	0·30
Silicone rubber point	1·10	0·45	1·00

Note: Higher values indicate rougher surfaces.

tobacco tars. The microfilled products are capable of retaining a smoother surface and are therefore more resistant to surface staining.

Cavity linings Although monomers employed in composite materials may be considered potentially harmful to the pulp, they are generally strongly bound in a highly cross-linked network following setting. Despite this, it is normal practice to line cavities prior to placement of a composite restoration. The material of choice is normally a calcium hydroxide product. Manufacturers of composite materials deter operators from using eugenol-containing liners because of the possible, though not definitely proven, adverse effects that eugenol may have on the setting and colour stability of the resin.

Adhesion Composite resins do not form a durable bond with tooth substance. Retention of the material is generally achieved by using undercut cavities. This often involves removing significant quantities of sound tooth substance.

Methods of establishing a bond between composite resins and enamel or dentine are discussed in Chap. 24. Such techniques greatly increase the number of potential applications of the materials and also offer a means of preventing microleakage.

Applications
Composite resins may be used as alternatives to silicate filling materials for the restoration of class III cavities. Other applications, such as the restoration of fractured incisal edges, depend upon the use of special techniques in which adhesion between restorative material and tooth substance is achieved. These are discussed in Chap. 24.

There is a growing tendency to consider composite resins for use as alternatives to amalgam in posterior cavities. Materials are available which appear to match amalgam in terms of physical properties, however, the technique of placement for composites in posterior teeth, without incorporating voids, is difficult. In addition, the durability of composites appears to be inferior to that of amalgam, particularly in class II cavities where considerable loss of anatomical form can take place due to wear. For class I cavities, where the material is fully surrounded by enamel, the wear is less noticeable.

There is some question over which group of composite materials offers the best chance of success in posterior teeth. Some clinical trials report encouraging results for microfilled composites after a year or two. They appear to wear rapidly following this early period of stability however, probably due to a fatigue process. Many of the products offered commercially as alternatives to amalgam are hybrid materials, particularly the light-activated variety. Materials containing barium glass fillers are most promising since they are radiopaque. They offer the practitioner the chance to confirm that the cavity has been correctly filled and also to check for the presence of caries in the surrounding dentine at subsequent examinations.

24 Adhesive Restorative Materials

24.1 Introduction

The development and regular use of adhesive materials has begun to revolutionize many aspects of restorative and preventive dentistry. Attitudes towards cavity preparation are altering since, with adhesive materials, it is no longer necessary to produce large undercuts in order to retain the filling. These techniques are, therefore, responsible for the conservation of large quantities of sound tooth substance which would otherwise be victim to the dental bur. Microleakage, a major dental problem which is probably responsible for many cases of secondary caries, may be reduced or eliminated. New forms of treatment, such as the sealing of pits and fissures on posterior teeth, the coverage of badly stained or deformed teeth in order to improve appearance and the direct bonding of brackets in orthodontics, have all grown from the development of adhesive systems.

Section 2.5 deals briefly with the general mechanistic aspects of adhesion. Two major approaches can be identified. Firstly, bonding through micro-mechanical attachment; in dentistry this is best illustrated through the bonding of resins to enamel using the *acid-etch technique*. Secondly, bonding through *chemical adhesion* to either enamel or dentine can be identified in many systems based on the use of coupling agents or cements containing polyacids.

24.2 Acid-etch systems for bonding to enamel

The surface of enamel is smooth and has little potential for bonding by micromechanical attachment. On treatment with certain acids, however, the structure of the enamel surface may be modified considerably. Fig. 24.1 shows the surface of human enamel following one minute of etching with a 30–50 percent solution of phosphoric acid, which is the acid of choice for most applications of the acid-etch technique.

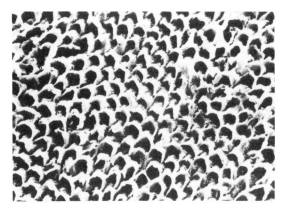

Fig. 24.1 Scanning electron microscope photograph of an enamel surface following one minute of etching with 37 percent aqueous phosphoric acid solution. (× 750)

The individual features evident in Fig. 24.1 correspond to the ends of enamel prisms, each being about 5 μm in diameter. This surface is now suitable for micromechanical attachment since it contains a myriad of small undercuts into which resins can gain ingress, set and form a 'mechanical lock'. The three major factors which affect the success or failure of acid-etch bonding systems are:

(1) The etching time. This should be sufficient to cause effective etching as evidenced by a white, chalky appearance on the treated section of enamel. Etching should not continue long enough for dissolved apatites to reprecipitate as phosphates onto the etched surface. The etching time normally used is between 10 and 60 seconds,

(2) The washing stage. Following etching the enamel surface should be washed with copious amounts of water to remove debris,

(3) The drying stage. The surface of the etched enamel should be very thoroughly dried using oil-free compressed air and maintained in a dry, uncontaminated state prior to application of the resin.

The type of resin applied to the etched enamel

surface depends upon the specific application being used. For composite resins the mixed material may be applied directly to the etched enamel surface. Resin from the composite flows into the etched enamel and sets, forming rigid tags, typically 25 μm long, which retain the filling. Many manufacturers supply a fluid *bonding resin* which may enhance the adhesive bond strength. It consists of a resin similar to that used in the composite material but contains no filler particles. It is very fluid and readily flows into the etched enamel surface. The bonding resin may be a single component which is activated by light or may consist of two fluid resins, one containing initiator and the other activator, which require mixing before being applied to the etched enamel. The composite resin filling material is applied directly to the surface of the bonding resin.

Although adequate bonding can be achieved with a composite resin alone, some practitioners prefer the 'extra security' which accrues from using an intermediate bonding resin.

Applications The acid-etch technique has many applications in dentistry. It is now widely used for most composite resin fillings as a means of reducing or preventing microleakage. For *class IV cavities* the acid-etch technique has replaced the gold inlay as the treatment of choice for restoring the tooth contours and function. In this example the use of an adhesive system allows the conservation of considerable quantities of tooth substance which would otherwise be lost in cavity preparation.

Fissure sealants, which are chemically similar to the bonding agents used to enhance adhesion, are now widely used for preventing pit and fissure caries.

Resin systems are now widely used for attaching *orthodontic brackets*. These resins are normally supplied as two components carrying relatively high loadings of initiator and activator respectively. One component is painted onto the etched enamel surface and the other onto the bracket. When the two are pressed together, rapid setting takes place.

$$- CH_2 - CH - CH_2 - CH - CH_2 - CH - CH_2 - \text{ etc.}$$

with CO_2H groups on the CH carbons

(a)

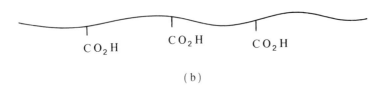

(b)

Fig. 24.2 Structural formula of polyacrylic acid and its cross-linking through zinc ions. (a) Polyacrylic acid. (b) Polyacrylic acid (simplified structural formula). (c) Simplified structural formula of polyacrylic acid cross-linked with zinc ions.

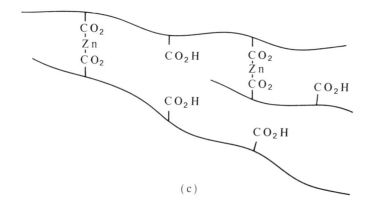

(c)

Alternatively, conventional composite resin materials can be used for this application.

Composite resins are gaining in popularity for the attachment of *bridges*. This is a more conservative technique than the traditional methods, which involve considerable destruction of the abutment teeth in order to achieve retention.

Another application is the attachment of acrylic *laminate veneers*, using the acid-etch technique and composite resin as the adhesive, as a means of improving the appearance of badly stained or misshapen teeth.

24.3 Bonding to dentine

It is recognized by most authorities that acid-etching should be restricted to use only on enamel surfaces. It has been demonstrated that acid treatment of dentine exposes the open ends of dentinal tubules, forming sites for possible mechanical retention. It is feared, however, that such treatment may cause irreparable damage to the dental pulp and, generally, is avoided. Indeed, during forms of treatment which involve etching of enamel, it is normally advised that exposed dentine should first be covered with a protective cavity base, normally a calcium hydroxide material.

Attempts to form adhesive bonds with dentine involve the use of materials containing *polyacrylic acid* or similar polyacid or the use of *coupling*

Table 24.1 Composition of glass ionomer cements

Powder/liquid materials

Powder	Sodiumaluminosilicate glass with about 20 percent CaF and other minor additives.
Liquid	Aqueous solution of acrylic acid/itaconic acid polymer.
or	Aqueous solution of maleic acid/acrylic acid copolymer.
or	Aqueous solution of maleic acid copolymer. Tartaric acid in some products to control setting characteristics.

Powder/water materials

Powder	Glass (as above) + freeze-dried polyacid (acrylic, maleic or copolymers).
Water	Manufacturers supply a dropper bottle which the operator fills with water.
or	The manufacturer supplies a dilute aqueous solution or tartaric acid.

---

agents which are able to chemically link the tooth surface with a restorative resin.

Materials containing polyacids

Two groups of materials rely, for their setting reaction, on the rapid cross-linking of polyacrylic acid, polymaleic acid or copolymers of acrylic and maleic or acrylic and itaconic acids with certain cations.

Fig. 24.2 shows the structural formula of polyacrylic acid and part of the cross-linked reaction product which results from reaction with zinc oxide. Similar products may be produced by reaction with calcium and aluminium ions.

Bonding of the materials to teeth is probably by reaction of carboxylic acid groups with calcium of tooth substance. This view is substantiated by the fact that higher tensile bond strengths can be achieved with enamel than with dentine which contains less inorganic material.

Polycarboxylate cements These materials may be supplied as a powder and liquid or as a powder which is mixed with water. For powder/liquid materials, the powder is finely ground zinc oxide which sometimes contains minor quantities of other oxides such as magnesium oxide. The liquid is an aqueous solution of polyacrylic of about 40 percent concentration. In the powder/water materials the powder contains zinc oxide and freeze-dried polyacrylic acid. On mixing the powder with water, the polyacrylic acid dissolves and starts to react with zinc oxide. The materials are primarily used as luting cements for attaching crowns, bridges and inlays or as cavity base materials. These applications are discussed in Chap. 29. The adhesive properties of the materials are occasionally utilized for the attachment of *orthodontic bands* since the material forms a strong bond with stainless steel as well as with enamel and dentine.

Glass ionomer cements (polyalkenoates)

Composition These materials, like the polycarboxylate cements, may be supplied as a powder and liquid or as a powder mixed with water. The composition is outlined in Table 24.1.

For powder/liquid materials the powder consists of a sodium aluminosilicate glass of similar composition to that used in silicate materials (p. 134) The ratio of alumina to silica in the glass is increased compared to that used in silicates. This

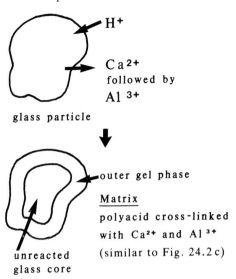

H⁺

Ca²⁺
followed by
Al³⁺

glass particle

outer gel phase

Matrix
polyacid cross-linked
with Ca²⁺ and Al³⁺
(similar to Fig. 24.2 c)

unreacted
glass core

Fig. 24.3 Schematic representation of the reaction of aluminosilicate glass particles with aqueous polyacid solutions.

increases the reactivity of the glass to a level where it reacts rapidly with polyacrylic acid, which is a much weaker acid than the phosphoric acid used in silicate materials. As for the silicates the glasses contain significant levels of fluoride which, although not directly involved in the setting reaction, has a significant effect on the caries susceptibility of the surrounding tooth substance.

The liquid component may consist of an aqueous solution of an acrylic acid/itaconic acid copolymer or of a maleic acid/acrylic acid copolymer. Tartaric acid, which is used to control setting characteristics, is also included in the liquid component by many manufacturers.

The powder/water materials are of two types. Both consist of a powder which contains freeze-dried polyacid, in addition to the glass powder. For some materials this is mixed with water and the manufacturers supply a dropper bottle to aid proportioning. With other products, the manufacturer supplies a dilute aqueous solution of tartaric acid. Some products are now available in encapsulated form.

Setting reaction Whichever material is used, on mixing the powder and liquid or powder and water the acid slowly degrades the outer layers of the glass particles releasing Ca^{2+} and Al^{3+} ions. During the early stages of setting, Ca^{2+} is released more

rapidly and is primarily responsible for reacting with the polyacid to form a reaction product akin to that shown in Fig. 24.2c. Al^{3+} is released more slowly and becomes involved in setting at a later stage, often referred to as a secondary reaction stage. These processes are illustrated in Fig. 24.3. The set material consists of unreacted glass cores embedded in a matrix of cross-linked polyacid. The reaction has many similarities with that discussed for silicate materials on p. 134.

Two types of glass ionomer material are available. Type I products are used for luting and cavity lining and are discussed in Chap. 29. The type II products are used as filling materials.

Properties Apart from the advantage of adhesion, which accrues from the reaction between polyacids and calcium of tooth substance, the properties of glass ionomer filling materials are similar to those of the silicates. The similarities with silicates extend to the handling characteristics and the special precautions required to achieve optimum properties. The powder/liquid ratio should be high in order to optimize strength and solubility but there should be sufficient free polyacid available to form a bond with tooth substance. The materials are often difficult to mix at the ratios recommended. The use of cooled mixing slabs helps and the powder/water materials tend to be easier to handle than the powder/liquid products. Aqueous solutions of polyacids should not be stored in a refrigerator since this may initiate crystallization.

The setting reaction is rather protracted despite a fairly rapid initial hardening. The material must be protected from moisture contamination during the first hour, otherwise strength and solubility are adversely affected. Hence it is necessary to varnish the surface of the filling immediately after initial hardening.

There is an important difference between glass ionomer materials and silicates in terms of biocompatibility. Although the glass ionomers are acidic they are far less irritant than silicates, for two reasons. Firstly, the acids used are much weaker acids than phosphoric acid. Secondly, the polyacid chains are very large and probably unable to pass down dentinal tubules. Only in very deep cavities having a thin residual layer of dentine is it considered necessary to use a cavity lining. In these cases, the lining of choice is normally one of the calcium hydroxide materials.

The glass ionomers are relatively brittle and cannot be considered suitable as general-purpose

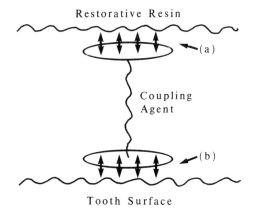

Restorative Resin

Coupling
Agent

(a)

(b)

Tooth Surface

Fig. 24.4 Diagram illustrating the principle of bonding with a coupling agent. (a) Part of molecule which enters into bonding with restorative resin. (b) Part of molecule which enters into bonding with tooth surface.

filling materials but more to answer a specific need for certain applications. The brittleness of the material, for example, would preclude the use of these products for restoring fractured incisal edges.

In terms of appearance, the materials are more translucent than the polycarboxylate cements since they contain considerable quantities of unreacted glass cores. They do not compare well with silicate materials however, being more opaque and less lifelike.

Applications The major applications of the glass ionomer filling materials reflect the advantages of adhesion coupled with a less than perfect aesthetic quality. They are widely used for restoring *abrasion cavities* normally occurring near the gingival margins of canine, premolar and molar teeth. Such cavities normally arise due to overzealous brushing combined with the use of an abrasive dentifrice. The cavities are often dish-shaped, caries-free and extend into the dentine in an area of the tooth where the thickness of dentine is minimal. The use of an adhesive material in these circumstances is most beneficial. After cleaning and drying the cavity, the mixed material may be applied directly with no cavity preparation apart from a finishing edge, sufficient retention accruing from the

adhesive bond. Fluoride release from the set material helps to retain the surrounding tooth substance in good order.

Glass ionomer cements are gaining wide acceptance as all-purpose filling materials for *deciduous teeth*. They allow the trauma of cavity preparation to be reduced to a minimum and, although they are probably not durable enough to withstand forces of mastication in adults, they are probably adequate for the limited life of deciduous teeth.

Another suggested use of glass ionomers is as *fissure sealants*. The material is mixed to a more fluid consistency to allow flow into the depths of the pits and fissures of posterior teeth.

The direct attachment of *orthodontic bands* is another suggested application.

Luting and cavity lining applications are covered in Chap. 29.

Adhesion promoters are often advocated for use with glass ionomers. Some manufacturers supply a citric acid solution which is used for pretreating the dentine surface prior to application of the material. This may thoroughly clean the surface and allow more efficient bond formation. The efficacy of citric acid pretreatment has been questioned, however, and it is thought that little benefit is gained. Other pretreatments including the use of hydrogen peroxide solution, polyacrylic acid solution and various types of remineralizing solutions have also been suggested.

Resin coupling agents
Resin-based restorative materials may be bonded to either dentine or enamel using coupling agents. The principle of the coupling agent is that it consists of a difunctional molecule, one part of which enters into chemical union with the tooth surface whilst the other attaches to the resin, as illustrated in Fig. 24.4. The method of use is to apply the coupling agent to the clean, dry tooth surface followed by the resin filling material, normally a composite.

One of the earliest molecules to be used for this purpose was *N*-phenylglycine–glycidylmethacrylate, NPG–GMA (Fig. 24.5). A complex bond is

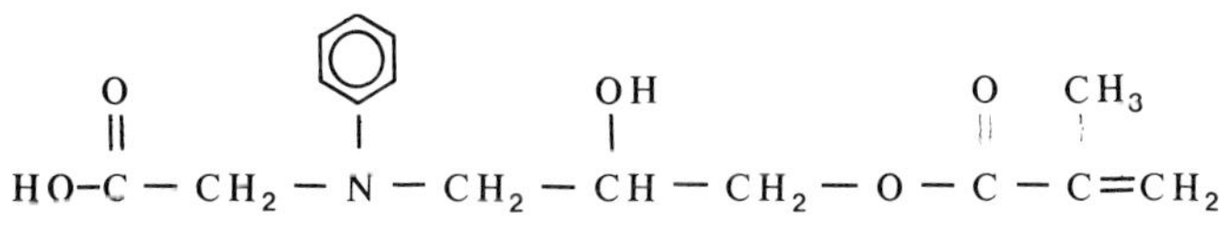

$$HO-\underset{\underset{O}{\|}}{C}-CH_2-\underset{H}{\underset{|}{N}}-CH_2-\underset{H}{\underset{|}{CH}}-CH_2-O-\underset{\underset{O}{\|}}{C}-\underset{\underset{CH_3}{|}}{C}=CH_2$$

Fig. 24.5 Structural formula of *N*-phenyl-glycine–glycidylmethacrylate (NPG–GMA). Used as a coupling agent to link composite resin restorative materials with tooth substance.

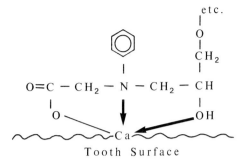

etc.

Fig. 24.6 Diagram illustrating the probable mechanism of adhesion between NPG–GMA and the tooth surface.

Table 24.2 Tensile bond strengths obtained between various restorative materials and tooth substance

Bonding couple	Bond strength (MPa)
Composite resin + acid-etched enamel	16·0
Composite resin + coupling agent + acid-etched enamel	21·0
Composite resin + coupling agent + dentine	5·0
Glass ionomer + enamel	5·0
Glass ionomer + dentine	3·5

formed between the *N*-phenylglycine group and the calcium of the tooth (Fig. 24.6), whilst the methacrylate group becomes incorporated into the resin during polymerization.

Other systems have been introduced more recently but are based on a similar principle. One product, for example, consists of a modified Bis GMA monomer with phosphate groups capable of forming a bond with tooth substance.

The coupling agents developed to date rely, mainly, on bonding to the mineral component of tooth substance. They therefore produce a higher bond strength with enamel than with dentine. Also, when bonding to dentine, the use of a cavity lining must be considered. Some manufacturers advocate the need for a protective lining in the deeper parts of dentine whilst others claim no lining is necessary.

When bonding to enamel, it is possible to use a combination of mechanical retention through acid-etching with chemical adhesion, using a coupling agent to give optimum bond strengths.

24.4 Comparative bond strengths

Table 24.2 gives values of tensile bond strengths obtained with various systems. The highest bond strengths are achieved using acid-etch systems and coupling agents in combination with a composite resin. Although the bond strengths achieved with glass ionomer materials appear much lower, examination of fracture surfaces reveals that fracture of the material–tooth bond often occurs cohesively through the glass ionomer material, indicating that the tensile bond strength is greater than the tensile strength of the material. For acid-etch systems without coupling agent, fracture normally occurs across the necks of the resin tags which produce the mechanical retention. When a coupling agent is used in combination with acid-etching, cohesive failure within the body of the resin may be observed on fracture surfaces. It appears that the bond strength values reported are approaching the optimum for the materials currently available.

Temporary Crown and Bridge Resins

25.1 Introduction

Temporary crown and bridge resins are used to provide immediate temporary coverage following tooth preparation for crowns or bridges.

The usual technique is to record an initial impression in an alginate material prior to tooth preparation. The major impression may be recorded then or subsequently using an elastomeric impression material. The mixed temporary crown or bridge resin is applied to the prepared areas by placing it into the desired area of the alginate impression which is reseated in the patient's mouth. After initial setting, the impression and the resin are removed and final hardening occurs outside the mouth. Temporary crowns can also be fabricated by placing the resins on to prepared teeth in clear plastic crown formers. In addition, the fit of prefabricated crowns can be improved by relining them with one of the temporary crown and bridge resins.

The temporary crowns and bridges are cemented into place with temporary cements, normally of a zinc oxide−eugenol composition.

25.2 Requirements

The product should ideally be non-injurious to oral tissues since it comes into direct contact with freshly cut dentine and the oral mucosa. During setting, it should not give an unduly large temperature rise whilst in contact with dentine, as this could damage the pulp. It should not undergo a large setting contraction which could make removal of the temporary crown or bridge difficult, particularly if the set material is rigid.

The material should also have convenient setting characteristics, including:

(1) Sufficient working time to allow mixing, placement into the impression and seating into the mouth,

(2) After seating in the mouth, rapid attainment of a 'rubbery' stage which facilitates its easy removal without distortion,

(3) Rapid hardening outside the mouth, enabling the trimmed crown or bridge to be cemented into place after a short time.

It should be strong and tough enough to resist fracture and wear in use and should, ideally, be tooth-coloured. Factors which affect durability and appearance are not of prime importance in view of the temporary nature of its use.

25.3 Available materials

Four types of material are available, as outlined in Table 25.1. The acrylic material is essentially identical with that discussed on p. 138 as a restorative resin.

The higher methacrylate resin is similar in many ways to the product sometimes used as a reline material for dentures and described on p. 92.

The epimine product is chemically similar to the epimines used in polyether impression materials (p. 122). In this case the central unit of the difunctional imine monomer (Fig. 19.7a) is aromatic in nature in order to produce a rigid polymer.

The composite material is different from those used as filling materials, which are not suitable for temporary crown and bridgework due to their unfavourable setting characteristics.

25.4 Properties

Setting characteristics Both the epimine resin and composite material have the advantage of exhibiting a distinct rubbery stage, during which the temporary crown or bridge can be removed from the patient's mouth without distortion or damage.

This rubbery phase is achieved in the composite material by the use of a multifunctional acrylic

Table 25.1 Temporary crown and bridge resins

Type	Dispensation method		Composition
Acrylic	Powder/liquid	Powder	Polymethylmethacrylate beads + peroxide
		Liquid	Methylmethacrylate monomer + activator
Higher methacrylate	Powder/liquid	Powder	Polyethylmethacrylate beads + peroxide
		Liquid	Isobutylmethacrylate + activator
Epimine	Paste/liquid	Paste	Imine-terminated prepolymer + polyamide filler
		Liquid	Sulphonic acid ester (reaction initiator)
Composite	3 Pastes	Base paste	Multifunctional methacrylic acid ester monomer + filler
		2 Catalyst pastes	One containing initiator, other containing activator

monomer which produces a relatively high cross-link density early on in the setting reaction. Normal filling composites do not possess this characteristic and set rapidly to a hard rigid solid.

After removing the epimine or composite crown during its rubbery stage, final setting can be accelerated by immersion in hot water for a few seconds.

The two types of acrylic material do pass through a rubbery stage, when removal is facilitated, but this stage is not as distinct as in the other two products.

None of the materials should be allowed to set completely *in situ* since they all undergo a significant setting contraction. This is greatest for the polymethylmethacrylate material where a volumetric shrinkage of about 5 percent occurs.

Each of the materials exhibits an exothermic reaction on setting, the temperature rise being greatest in the acrylic material. This may have important biological consequences, when a considerable bulk of resin is present, in constructing a large temporary crown or bridge on freshly cut vital dentine. One should ensure that the materials are removed from the patient's mouth well before their maximum temperature rise has occurred. This relies on being able to identify the commencement of the rubbery stage after which the maximum temperature is normally reached within a minute or two.

Biocompatibility Certain components of some of the products are known to have an irritant effect when placed on freshly cut vital dentine. Methylmethacrylate monomer, for example, present in the

acrylic material, falls into this category. When using this product it is necessary to either varnish the preparations or apply a surface layer of petroleum jelly as a protective measure. The isobutylmethacrylate monomer used in the higher methacrylate product is far less irritant than methylmethacrylate. The sulphonic acid ester catalyst present in the epimine material occasionally causes irritation of soft tissues adjacent to the prepared teeth and a degree of protection may be afforded by coating such tissues with a layer of petroleum jelly.

Mechanical properties The mechanical properties of the materials become most significant when minimal tooth tissue removal or shoulderless crown preparations are used. There is a danger of fracture occurring in the thin areas at the tapered margin of such a temporary crown. This is most likely in the acrylic material which is weaker and more brittle than the other products.

Appearance In terms of appearance the acrylic, higher methacrylate and epimine materials have an advantage in that they are available in a range of shades and a good match with tooth substance can be achieved. The composite material is available as a 'universal' shade.

26

Requirements of Dental Cements

26.1 Introduction

Cements are widely used in dentistry for a variety of applications. Some products are used primarily for *cavity lining* whilst others are primarily used for *luting* applications. Other, more specialist products, are used for sealing root canals as part of a course of *endodontic treatment*.

26.2 Requirements of cavity lining materials

Certain filling materials are not suitable for placing directly into a freshly prepared cavity. In such circumstances, a layer of cavity lining material is placed in the base of the cavity, and on the axial dentine wall for class II cavities, prior to placement of the filling. The requirements of the cavity lining material chosen for any specific application depend on the *depth of the cavity*, which determines the *thickness of residual dentine* between the base of the cavity and the dental pulp, and the *type of filling material* which is being used to restore the tooth.

The purpose of the cavity lining, or *cavity base*, is to act as a barrier between the filling material and the dentine which, by virtue of the dentinal tubules, has direct access to the sensitive pulp. Depending upon the specific circumstances, the lining may be expected to provide a *thermal, chemical* and *electrical* barrier as illustrated in Fig. 26.1.

A thermally insulating cavity lining is required when a metallic filling, such as amalgam, or a filling which sets by a highly exothermic reaction, such as acrylic resin, is used. Table 21.3 shows that the thermal diffusivity value for amalgam is about 40 times greater than that for dentine. In deep cavities, having only a thin residual layer of dentine, there is a danger of 'thermal shock' to the pulp when the patient takes hot or cold food. A layer of insulating cavity lining material of sufficient thickness helps to prevent this. In shallow

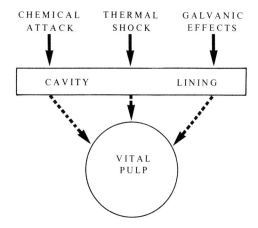

Fig. 26.1 Diagram illustrating the way in which a cavity lining protects the dental pulp.

cavities, where there is a relatively thick layer of residual dentine, it becomes less important to use a lining with thermal insulating properties. Indeed, for amalgam restorations in shallow cavities, the use of a thick layer of cavity lining may reduce the thickness of the overlying amalgam to such an extent that it becomes weakened and liable to fracture. Hence, in such shallow cavities, the base and walls of the cavity are generally lined with a *varnish*. This consists of a solution of a natural or synthetic resin in a volatile solvent. It is painted into the cavity and the solvent evaporates to leave a very thin layer of resin which helps to seal the ends of the dentinal tubules. The varnishes do not provide adequate thermal protection in deep cavities since they form only a thin layer.

Cavity lining materials are sometimes required to form a protective barrier against potential chemical irritants present in some filling materials. Phosphoric acid in silicate materials, and acrylic monomers in some resin-based materials, are two such potential irritants.

When an amalgam restoration is placed adjacent to, or opposing, a gold restoration it is possible to set up a galvanic cell which not only accelerates corrosion but can cause pain. The use of an electrically insulating lining material helps to prevent such activity. Unfortunately, most of the lining materials used are either water-based or contain polar organometallic compounds. They are not, therefore, ideal electrical insulators. Varnishes consisting of less polar resins, such as polystyrene, may be used to provide some electrical resistance. These are sometimes painted onto the surface of metallic

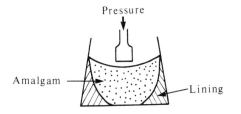

Fig. 26.2 Flow of an unset cement lining caused by the high pressure of condensation.

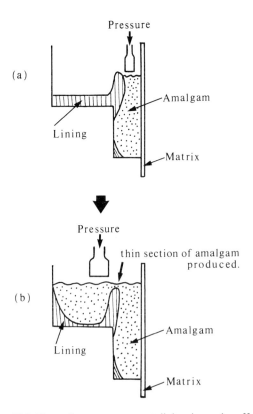

Fig. 26.3 Flow of an unset cement lining in a class II cavity caused by the high pressure of condensation. (a) Whilst filling the box. (b) Whilst filling the occlusal part of the cavity.

restorations giving temporary relief to the symptoms of 'galvanic pain'.

The biological properties of the lining material itself are important. The products used should, ideally, be non-irritant and possess bacteriostatic properties.

The vast majority of cavity lining materials are supplied as two components which are mixed together, initiating a setting reaction. The setting characteristics should allow sufficient time for mixing and placing in the cavity followed by rapid setting in order that the filling material can be placed without too much delay.

The lining should remain intact during the placement of the filling material. The integrity of the lining depends on several factors, for example:

(1) The degree of set achieved at the time the filling material is placed,

(2) The strength of the set material and its thickness,

(3) The type of cavity,

(4) The pressure exerted during the placement of the filling material,

(5) The degree of support from surrounding structures,

(6) The choice of correct operative techniques.

If the lining is not set, when amalgam condensation commences for example, there is every possibility that the material will undergo considerable flow due to the high pressures used. This is illustrated in Fig. 26.2 for a class I cavity and 26.3 for a class II cavity. It can be seen that in both cases the insulating layer of lining is lost and the amalgam comes into close contact with dentine. For the class II cavity, a further danger is the production of a thin section of amalgam as the lining flows upwards during the packing of the interproximal box (Fig. 26.3a) and is forced further upwards during the filling of the remainder of the cavity (Fig. 26.3b).

If the lining material has set at the time of amalgam condensation there is little chance of flow. The strength of the set material should be sufficient to resist fracture. For class I cavities there is little chance of fracturing a set lining, even though it may have relatively low strength, since it is supported on all sides by a rigid cocoon of tooth substance (Fig. 26.4). For class II cavities the situation is different, as illustrated in Fig. 26.5. The axial wall of lining is unsupported and attempts to condense amalgam directly onto this may cause fracture at the exposed corner. This technique not only destroys the integrity of the lining but may

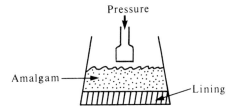

Fig. 26.4 There is little danger of fracturing a cement lining in a class I cavity since it is fully supported by dentine on all sides.

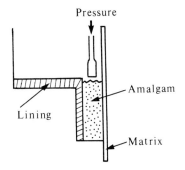

Fig. 26.6 The problem highlighted in Fig. 26.5 is overcome by condensing amalgam into the interproximal box first. This then provides support for the cement lining of the axial wall and the occlusal part of the cavity can be filled without causing fracture.

produce an incompletely filled cavity, having voids as shown.

The correct technique is to condense amalgam into the interproximal box first, as shown in Fig. 26.6. This provides support for the lining of the axial wall which can then withstand direct forces.

The placement of other filling materials does not present problems as severe as those encountered with amalgam condensation since much smaller forces are used for adaptation. If the lining material is properly set, there is little chance of flow and fracture is also unlikely at lower pressures.

Cavity linings should, ideally, be radiopaque in order that the dentist can observe them on radiographs, thereby aiding the diagnosis of caries around the filling. A radiolucent lining material may hinder the early detection of such lesions.

Finally, the cavity lining material chosen for any particular application must be compatible with the filling material which is placed above it. The constituents of the lining should not have any effect on the setting characteristics or properties of the filling.

26.3 Requirements of luting materials

Many dental appliances and restorations are constructed outside the patient's mouth and then fixed into place using a cement luting material. Examples include the fixing of porcelain and metal crowns, bridges, inlays and metal posts.

Many of the requirements of luting materials are similar to those of cavity lining materials, for example, the material should, ideally, be non-irritant. This requirement is not as critical for luting as for cavity lining since the luting cement is normally applied to a thicker residual layer of dentine than would exist in a deep cavity.

The *setting characteristics* should allow sufficient time for mixing the material, applying to the restoration and/or tooth preparation and for seating the restoration in place in the mouth. The material should, ideally, be of low initial viscosity or be pseudoplastic, to allow flow of the cement lute so

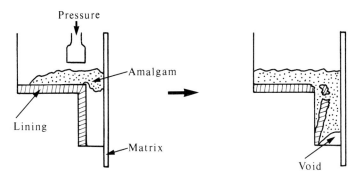

Fig. 26.5 When condensing amalgam into a class II cavity, the cement lining on the axial wall is most vulnerable to fracture.

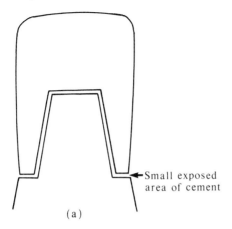

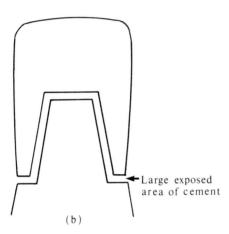

Fig. 26.7 The thickness of the cement lute may vary according to the viscosity of the cement at the time of seating the restoration. (a) Thin layer of cement. (b) Thicker layer of cement.

that proper seating can occur. If the viscosity of the cement is high at the time of insertion there is a danger of the restoration being incompletely seated. For crowns, a thick layer of cement is produced at the margins as illustrated in Fig. 26.7. An indication of the ability of a cement to flow during seating is sometimes obtained by measurements of *film thickness*. A given volume of mixed cement is placed on a flat surface and at a predetermined time is compressed under a constant load. The thickness of the film of cement produced gives an indication of the flow during seating of a crown or other restoration.

Luting cements should, ideally, give thermal and electrical *insulation* since many of the restorations commonly cemented to teeth are based on alloys,

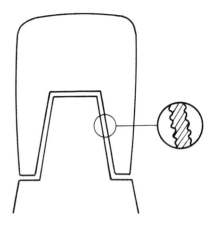

Fig. 26.8 Diagram illustrating how the cement lute gives mechanical retention of the restoration by entering small interstices in the tooth and restoration surface.

for example gold crowns.

The *retention* of restorations depends on the correct design and accuracy of the restoration and on the strength of the cement. Fig. 26.8 illustrates how the cement enters microscopic interstices on the rough tooth and restoration surface. On setting, the cement gives mechanical resistance to the displacement of the restoration, and must be strong enough to resist fracture when loads are applied to the restoration. Retention may be further improved if the luting cement chemically adheres to the tooth surface and restoration.

The *solubility* of a luting cement should be low because cement margins are often exposed to oral fluids as illustrated in Fig. 26.7. Dissolution or erosion of the cement may lead to failure by loss of retention or by the initiation of caries in the tooth substance adjacent to the eroded lute.

26.4 Requirements of endodontic cements
Certain forms of treatment require removal of the pulp followed by sterilization of the root canal. The cleaned canal is then filled with a silver, gutta-percha or silicone rubber point which is normally retained using a cement sealer. Alternative forms of treatment involve the sealing of the canal with cement sealer alone, but this is not a widely used or recommended procedure.

The requirements of the cement sealer are mainly concerned with its biocompatibility and its ability to resist dissolution and to form a good seal, both along the walls and at the apex of the canal.

The material should also be radiopaque in order that the dentist can confirm the attainment of a satisfactory root filling radiographically.

Cements used for sealing root canals must have setting characteristics which enable them to be forced into the warm, moist environment of the root canal before setting. This would not be possible with some conventional cements which set almost instantaneously in the presence of moisture. Hence, specialist products have been developed for endodontic applications.

Cements Based on Phosphoric Acid

27.1 Introduction

One group of widely used cements is based on the vigorous reaction which occurs between certain basic oxides and phosphoric acid to form phosphate salts of low solubility. The three products considered in this section are the *zinc phosphate* cements, *silicophosphate* cements and *copper phosphate* cements. The *silicate* filling materials described in Chap. 22 are closely related, having a liquid component which is essentially an aqueous solution of phosphoric acid and a powder which is a glass derived from amphoteric or basic oxides, but these are considered separately due to their different applications.

27.2 Zinc phosphate cements

Composition These materials are generally supplied as a powder and liquid which are mixed together by hand. Encapsulated products are available but are rarely used due to the extra cost involved.

The compositions of powder and liquid in a typical cement are given in Table 27.1. The major reactive component of the powder is zinc oxide. Small quantities of other oxides such as magnesium oxide may also be present. The liquid is essentially an aqueous solution of phosphoric acid buffered by adding small quantities of zinc oxide or aluminium oxide. These compounds form phosphates which

stabilize the pH of the acid and reduce its reactivity.

Setting reaction On mixing the powder and liquid together a vigorous reaction occurs, resulting in the formation of a relatively insoluble zinc phosphate as follows:

$$3ZnO + 2H_3PO_4 + H_2O \rightarrow Zn_3(PO_4)_2 \cdot 4H_2O$$

Only the surface layers of the zinc oxide particles react, leaving unconsumed cores bound together by the phosphate matrix.

The reaction is rapid and exothermic although its rate is tempered somewhat by the presence of buffers in the acid and a special process of deactivation of the zinc oxide powder involving heating and sintering with other, less reactive oxides.

Manipulative variables The powder/liquid ratio depends on the application. For cavity lining a putty-like consistency having a powder/liquid ratio of about 3·5:1 is used. For luting, a more fluid mix, with lower powder/liquid ratio, is employed to ensure flow of the cement during seating of the restoration. It is not normal practice to measure the proportions of powder or liquid but rather to assess the suitability of the mix 'by experience'. When proportioning, it is important to remember that lowering the powder/liquid ratio produces a weaker, more soluble and more irritant material.

The powder is best incorporated into the liquid in small increments until the desired consistency is reached. Mixing is easier if carried out on a cooled

Table 27.1 Composition of zinc phosphate cements

Powder	Zinc oxide	Approximately 90 percent as main active ingredient.
	Other metallic oxides	Approximately 10 percent.
Liquid	Aqueous solution of phosphoric acid	50–60 percent concentration.
	$Al_3(PO_4)_2$ $Zn_3(PO_4)_2$	Up to 10 percent as buffers.

glass mixing slab. Care must be taken, however, not to cool the mixing slab below the dew point, since water may condense from the atmosphere into the mix of cement below this temperature. Excess water affects both the setting characteristics and the physical properties of the set material. Proportioning and mixing are greatly simplified by using pre-encapsulated materials. Some products are supplied pre-encapsulated in syringes which enable the mixed material to be syringed into place following mechanical mixing for 5 or 10 seconds.

For hand-mixed powder/liquid systems it is necessary to take precautions over the handling of the liquid. The cap should be removed from the liquid bottle only long enough to dispense sufficient liquid for one mix, and then replaced immediately. If the liquid is left open to the atmosphere for extended periods, water will either be lost or gained depending upon the ambient humidity. Such changes in the water content of the liquid may alter the setting characteristics and physical properties of the material.

When using the materials for luting, the working time is optimized by adding the cement to the fitting surface of the restoration, which is initially at room temperature, and not to the tooth preparations which are at mouth temperature (37°C). If the cement is added to the tooth preparations first, there is every chance that its viscosity will have increased considerably before the restoration can be seated. In extreme cases the cement may even be completely set. This demonstrates the marked effect of temperature on the rate of re-action for these products.

Properties Providing the materials are mani-pulated correctly, the phosphate cements have suf-ficient working time to allow placement of a cavity lining or cement lute before the viscosity has in-creased markedly. At the lower powder/liquid ratio used for luting, the material is sufficiently fluid to allow seating of the restoration and formation of a thin film of lute.

Initial hardening of the material normally occurs within 4−7 minutes, although the strength continues to increase for some time after that. The com-pressive strength ultimately reaches a value of about 80 MPa for luting cement and 140 MPa for lining material, reflecting the differing powder/liquid ratios used. For lining materials used beneath amalgam restorations, the mechanical pro-perties at between 3 and 6 minutes after placing are important, since this is the time at which amalgam

is normally condensed. This time has been reduced over the years by the increased use of mechanically mixed amalgams requiring only a few seconds tri-turation. At about 5 minutes after placement a typical zinc phosphate lining cement has a com-pressive strength of only 30 MPa. This value is comparable with the stress used by some practi-tioners during amalgam condensation. Fracture of lining is unlikely since it is almost totally constrained in both class I and class II cavities providing a correct technique is used, (Figs. 26.5 & 26.6). The materials have generally achieved a sufficient degree of set at 5 minutes to resist flow during amalgam condensation.

The set material has a small, though significant, solubility in water and cement lute margins may erode slowly in the mouth by a combination of dissolution and abrasion. The cement lute is, potentially, the weak link of any indirect resto-ration since it normally joins two resistant materials, for example, gold and enamel or dentine, or porcelain and dentine. Erosion, leading to loss of the cement lute and failure of the resto-ration, is not, however, a problem particularly associated with zinc phosphate cements. Loss of restorations is more likely to occur due to a poor retentive design of the restoration.

Zinc phosphate cements may have an irritant effect on the dental pulp, particularly when used as cavity lining materials. The pH value of the cement at the time of application to the tooth is between 2 and 4 depending on the particular brand and the powder/liquid ratio. The degree of irritation depends on the depth of the cavity and the thick-ness of residual dentine. Zinc phosphate cements are unsuitable for use as linings in deep cavities unless a sublining of a less irritant material such as calcium hydroxide cement or zinc oxide/eugenol cement is used (Fig. 28.3).

The phosphate materials have adequate thermal insulating properties when used under metallic restorations. The value of thermal diffusivity does not differ markedly from that of tooth substance. They are not able to form an effective chemical barrier, however, due to their inherent acidity.

The set material is opaque due to a high concen-tration of unreacted zinc oxide. This may detract from the aesthetic appeal of a porcelain crown having a zinc phosphate lute, particularly if the cement lute margin is visible.

Zinc phosphate cements are widely used for all types of luting applications, and as cavity linings under amalgam fillings.

27.3 Silicophosphate cements

Silicophosphate cements are, essentially, hybrids of zinc phosphate and silicate materials. They are supplied as a powder and liquid. The liquid is an aqueous solution of phosphoric acid, containing buffers, whilst the powder is, essentially, a mixture of zinc oxide and aluminosilicate glass. The setting reaction produces a matrix of zinc and aluminium phosphates enclosing unreacted cores of zinc oxide and glass particles.

The set material is less soluble and more translucent than zinc phosphate cement.

These materials are used, primarily, as luting cements for porcelain crowns, where their extra translucency at the margins is considered an advantage, and as temporary filling materials.

27.4 Copper cements

These materials are closely related to the zinc phosphate cements. They are supplied as a powder and liquid. The liquid is an aqueous solution of phosphoric acid whilst the powder is a mixture of zinc oxide and black copper oxide. The setting reaction is similar to that for zinc phosphate materials.

The two properties which distinguish these products from simple zinc phosphate materials are their black appearance and their bactericidal effects, produced by the presence of copper.

The materials are not widely used nowadays, although they can be used as filling materials in deciduous teeth where it has not been possible to remove all caries. Their durability is not good but they are capable of preserving such teeth until they exfoliate. Another application is the cementation of splints and orthodontic appliances, although they have been largely superceded by other materials for the latter application.

28

Cements Based on Organometallic Chelate Compounds

28.1 Introduction

Many cements used in dentistry can be characterized by setting reactions which involve the formation of chelate compounds between zinc ions and *ortho*-disubstituted aromatic compounds. Three types of aromatic compound are commonly used, delineating the three groups of materials as follows:

(1) Zinc oxide/eugenol cements,
(2) *Ortho*-ethoxybenzoic acid (EBA) cements,
(3) Calcium hydroxide cements, in which the aromatic ligands are salicylates.

28.2 Zinc oxide/eugenol cements

Composition and setting These products may be supplied as a powder and liquid or as two pastes. The composition of a typical powder/liquid material is given in Table 28.1. The small quantity of zinc acetate in the powder acts as an accelerator by helping to create an ionic medium in which the setting reaction can occur. Some commercial products contain hydrogenated rosin or polystyrene and are known as *resin-reinforced* zinc oxide/eugenol cements. The relative proportions of powder and liquid are not normally measured accurately, although some manufacturers provide a

scoop which gives a known volume of powder to which a given number of drops of liquid are added. Thin mixes, having a low powder/liquid ratio, should be avoided since they produce inferior properties — lower strength and higher solubility. The paste/paste materials are similar to the impression pastes described on p. 109. These have the advantage of easier proportioning and mixing.

The setting reaction involves chelation of two eugenol molecules (Fig. 17.2) with one zinc ion to form zinc eugenolate (Fig. 17.3). This reaction proceeds very slowly in the absence of moisture. When the mixed material contacts water, however, setting is often completed within a few seconds.

Properties The setting characteristics of the zinc oxide/eugenol cements are, to some extent, ideal. They offer a combination of adequate working time, during which very little increase in viscosity occurs, coupled with rapid setting after placing into the cavity. The latter is caused by residual moisture in the cavity and the higher temperature of the mouth compared to room temperature. The effect of cavity moisture is noteworthy, particularly since efforts are generally made to dry the cavity before placement of a lining. Only very small amounts of water are required to cause the accelerating effect.

The ultimate compressive strength values for the zinc oxide/eugenol cements are somewhat lower than those recorded for zinc phosphate materials, typically 20 MPa for unreinforced materials and 40 MPa for reinforced materials. The nature of the setting reaction is such, however, that the materials develop their strength rapidly and the reinforced materials in particular are unlikely to flow or fracture during amalgam condensation, providing correct technique is used.

Zinc oxide/eugenol cements may be used as linings in deep cavities without causing harm to the pulp. Unconsumed eugenol is able to leach from the set material and although this substance has

Table 28.1 Composition of zinc oxide/eugenol cements

	Component	Function
Powder	Zinc oxide	Primary reactive ingredient.
	Zinc acetate (1−5 percent)	Accelerator.
Liquid	Eugenol	Primary reactive ingredient.
	Olive oil (5−15 percent)	To control viscosity.

Table 28.2 Composition of an *ortho*-ethoxybenzoic acid (EBA) cement

	Component	Function
Powder	Zinc oxide (approximately 60 percent)	Primary reactive ingredient.
	Quartz (approximately 35 percent) Hydrogenated rosin (approximately 5 percent)	Reinforcing agents.
Liquid	O-ethoxybenzoic acid Eugenol	Reactive ingredients.

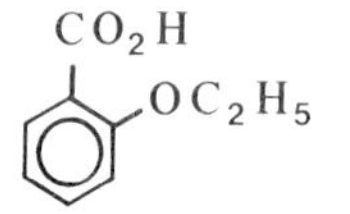

Fig. 28.1 Structural formula of *ortho*-ethoxybenzoic acid.

been shown to be irritant under certain conditions, it appears to have an obtundant effect on the pulp.

The ease with which eugenol can gain egress from the material is responsible for its relatively high solubility. Leached eugenol is replaced by water which, under certain conditions, can cause hydrolysis of the zinc eugenolate and disintegration of the cement structure. The materials are, therefore, not suitable for luting applications except on a temporary basis.

Free eugenol may also have an effect on resin-based filling materials, interfering with the polymerization process and sometimes causing discolouration. The materials are, therefore, not suitable as linings under this type of filling material.

The materials form an effective thermal barrier under metallic restorations having a value of thermal diffusivity similar to that for dentine.

The main uses of these cements are for linings under amalgam restorations, either used alone or as a sublining overlaid with a zinc phosphate material. They are also used as temporary luting cements and as temporary filling materials.

Root-canal pastes These pastes, used alone or in combination with a gutta-percha or silver point, are often modifications of zinc oxide/eugenol cavity lining materials. They contain additives, such as barium sulphate which render the materials radio-opaque, and small quantities of water-absorbing compounds which effectively increase the working times of the materials under moist conditions. Some materials contain therapeutic agents such as anti-inflammatory drugs and disinfectants. Para-formaldehyde is used as a disinfectant in some products, the utilization of which has been criticized because of the highly irritant effect which this substance can have on periapical tissues if the root filling inadvertently goes beyond the apex.

28.3 *Ortho*-ethoxybenzoic acid (EBA) cements

Composition These cements are generally supplied as a powder and liquid. The composition of a typical material is given in Table 28.2. The ratio of *o*-ethoxybenzoic acid to eugenol in the liquid may vary from one product to another but is usually about 2:1. The structural formula of *o*-ethoxybenzoic acid is given in Fig. 28.1. Comparison with Fig. 17.2 shows the similarity between the structure of *o*-ethoxybenzoic acid and eugenol. Both compounds are able to form chelate compounds with zinc ions. The structural formula for zinc eugenolate is shown in Fig. 17.3. The structure of zinc *o*-ethoxybenzoate is very similar.

Properties and applications The setting characteristics are similar to those of the zinc oxide/eugenol materials and are similarly affected by moisture. It is possible to achieve a higher powder/liquid ratio with these products since much of the powder consists of inert, reinforcing filler.

The set material is significantly stronger than even the reinforced zinc oxide/eugenol products due to the high powder/liquid ratio and the presence of fillers. A typical commercial product has an ultimate compressive strength of around 85 MPa. In addition, the lower level of residual eugenol, coupled with a greater resistance to hydrolysis of the zinc *o*-ethoxybenzoate, produces a cement with

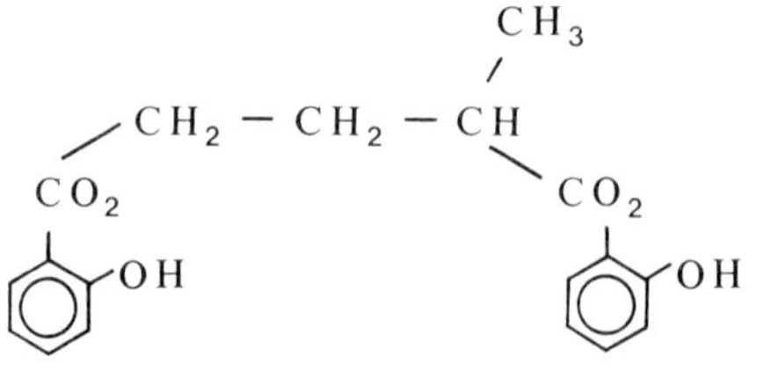

Fig. 28.2 Structural formula of butylene glycol disalicylate.

Table 28.3 Composition of a typical calcium hydroxide cement

	Component	Function
Paste 1	Calcium hydroxide (50 percent) Zinc oxide (10 percent)	Primary reactive ingredients.
	Zinc stearate (0·5 percent)	Accelerator.
	Ethyl toluene sulphonamide (39·5 percent)	Oily compound, acts as carrier.
Paste 2	Glycol salicylate (40 percent)	Primary reactive ingredient.
	Titanium dioxide Calcium sulphate Calcium tungstate	Inert fillers, pigments and radiopacifiers.

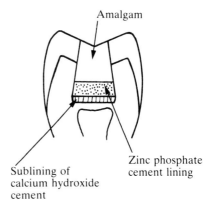

Fig. 28.3 Diagram showing the use of a calcium hydroxide cement as a sublining beneath a zinc phosphate cement lining.

lower solubility than that observed for zinc oxide/ eugenol products. Thermal characteristics are similar to those of the zinc oxide/eugenol materials.

The materials form a suitable cavity lining for amalgam condensation due to their adequate strength and resistance to flow, although they are primarily used as luting cements.

28.4 Calcium hydroxide cements

Composition Some calcium hydroxide preparations consist simply of a suspension of calcium hydroxide in water. This is applied to the base of the cavity and dries out to give a layer of calcium hydroxide. These materials are both difficult to manipulate and form a very friable cavity lining which is easily fractured. Most calcium hydroxide products in current use are supplied in the form of two components, normally pastes, which set following mixing to form a more substantial cavity lining. The composition of a typical commercial product is given in Table 28.3.

The structural formula of butylene glycol disalicylate, a glycol salicylate commonly used in one of the pastes, is given in Fig. 28.2. This is a difunctional chelating agent having two aromatic groups with reactive groups in *ortho* positions. On mixing this with a paste containing zinc oxide and calcium hydroxide, chelate compounds with structures similar to that shown in Fig. 17.3 are formed. It is thought that zinc ions are primarily responsible for chelation, with calcium being largely unreacted.

The sulphonamide compound used in the zinc oxide/calcium hydroxide paste is present merely as a carrier and is not thought to have any therapeutic effect.

Properties The mixed materials have very low viscosity and setting can be relatively slow for some products. Moisture has a dramatic effect on the rate of setting however, and the materials set within a few seconds of being placed in the cavity, even when the cavity has been 'dried'.

The set material is relatively weak compared to other cements, having a compressive strength of about 20 MPa. This strength is gained rapidly, however, and under the constrained conditions of a cavity the material is able to resist flow and fracture during amalgam condensation, providing correct technique is used.

The consistency of the materials makes them difficult to apply to cavities in thick section. In deep cavities, therefore, a commonly used technique is to apply a thin sublining of a calcium hydroxide cement and then to build up the base of the cavity with a zinc phosphate material prior to amalgam condensation, as illustrated in Fig. 28.3.

The set materials have a relatively high solubility in aqueous media. Calcium hydroxide is readily leached out, generating an alkaline environment in the area surrounding the cement. This is thought to be responsible for the proven antibacterial properties of these materials. This characteristic is utilized in very deep carious lesions, sometimes involving exposure of the pulp, or occasionally in cases of traumatic exposure of the pulp during cavity preparation. The calcium hydroxide cement is used as a *pulp capping* agent in such situations. It is sufficiently biocompatible to be placed adjacent to the pulp and capable of destroying any remaining bacteria. The material is also able to initiate calcification and formation of a secondary dentine layer at the base of the cavity. In pulp capping procedures the calcium hydroxide material is generally overlaid with a strong cement base material such as zinc phosphate cement before completing the restoration of the tooth with amalgam.

Calcium hydroxide cements are routinely used as lining materials beneath silicate and resin-based filling materials. Unlike the eugenol-containing cements they have no adverse effect on these filling materials and form an effective chemical barrier against acids and monomers.

Calcium hydroxide preparations, similar to those used for cavity lining and pulp capping but containing retarders, are now available as root-canal sealing pastes.

The high solubility and low strength of the calcium hydroxide cements render them unsuitable for luting purposes.

29

Cements Based on Polyalkenoic Acids

29.1 Introduction

Two types of cement based on polyacids are in common use for both luting and cavity lining applications. The first products to be developed were the *polycarboxylate* cements which rely on the reaction between zinc oxide and a polyacid. The second group of products are described as *glass ionomer* or *polyalkenoate* cements. The setting reaction takes place between a polyacid molecule and cations released from an ion-leachable glass.

29.2 Polycarboxylate cements

The composition, chemistry of setting, and adhesive properties of these products, are given on p. 149. Many recently developed products contain fluoride salts which exert an anticariogenic effect on surrounding tooth substance.

The cements have sufficient early strength to resist amalgam condensation and, allowing for product variations, have an ultimate compressive strength of about 80 MPa, a similar value to that recorded for the EBA materials.

The polycarboxylate materials are acidic, though not as irritant as phosphate cements, for two reasons. Polyacrylic acid is a weaker acid than phosphoric acid and the polyacid chains are too large and lack the mobility required to penetrate dentinal tubules. Despite the more biocompatible nature of these materials they are not widely used as linings in very deep cavities unless a sublining of a calcium hydroxide or zinc oxide/eugenol material is used.

Laboratory tests show that the solubility values of polycarboxylate cements are greater than those for the zinc phosphate, silicophosphate and glass ionomer materials. Despite this apparent disadvantage, the materials are widely used for luting without appearing to display an unduly high failure rate.

The materials form an adhesive bond with enamel and dentine but only a weak bond with gold and no perceptible bond with porcelain. Hence, the adhesive nature of the materials when used for the luting of gold or porcelain crowns is only utilized to a limited degree and cannot be considered an overwhelming advantage for such applications. The materials form a strong bond with stainless steel which makes them useful for attaching orthodontic bands. Care must be taken when using steel instruments for mixing and placing. Excess material should be removed from such instruments before it sets, otherwise a tenacious bond will form.

As for most other cements, strength and solubility are optimized by achieving a high powder/liquid ratio. For polycarboxylate materials however, two restricting factors should be remembered. Firstly, some free polyacid is required to form an adhesive bond and this will not be possible if a very dry mix is used. Secondly, a relatively low viscosity is required to allow seating of restorations during luting.

The set materials are opaque due to a high concentration of unreacted zinc oxide cores. This may detract from the appearance of porcelain crowns, particularly if the cement lute margin is visible.

29.3 Glass ionomer cements (polyalkenoates)

The use of glass ionomers as filling materials is discussed on p. 149. The cavity lining and luting cements are of broadly similar composition to that given in Table 24.1. One difference is that the luting and cavity lining cements contain glass of smaller particle size to allow the formation of a thinner film thickness during luting. Powder/liquid and powder/water materials are both available and widely used.

The set materials are stronger than the polycarboxylate products having a compressive strength value of about 130 MPa, although there may be wide variations from one product to another. The materials can withstand amalgam condensation and are occasionally used as cavity linings for amalgam restorations. Their biological properties are akin to those of the polycarboxylate cements which are covered in the previous section. Although they are considered relatively bland they are rarely used as linings in very deep cavities.

The glass ionomer cements are less soluble than the polycarboxylates, and most of the other cement products, when measured under ideal laboratory conditions. The solubility can be adversely affected by early moisture contamination, however, as discussed on p. 150 for the glass ionomer filling materials. It is essential that cement lute margins are covered with a layer of a protective varnish immediately after seating the restoration. This can often be a difficult procedure, particularly if the margins lie subgingivally. Although the glass ionomers are theoretically capable of producing an insoluble cement lute this ideal may not be easy to achieve in practice.

The materials display the same adhesive properties as the polycarboxylates and are more translucent due to the presence of unreacted cores of glass rather than zinc oxide. The extra translucency is considered an advantage for luting porcelain crowns, although further improvements in appearance are required if the cement is to be truly able to match porcelain.

Recommended Further Reading

COMBE E.C. (1981) *Notes on Dental Materials*, 4th Edition. Edinburgh: Churchill Livingstone.

CRAIG R.G. ed. (1978) *Dental Materials — A Problem Oriented Approach*. St Louis: C.V. Mosby Co.

CRAIG R.G. (1980) *Restorative Dental Materials*, 6th Edition. St Louis: C.V. Mosby Co.

PHILIPS R.W. (1973) *Skinner's Science of Dental Materials*, 7th Edition. Philadelphia: W.B Saunders.

Status reports on materials and techniques published by the Council on Dental Materials, Instruments and Equipment in association with the American Dental Association. These reports are published regularly in the *Journal of the American Dental Association*. e.g. State of the art and science of bonding in orthodontic treatment. *Journal of the American Dental Association*, vol. **105**, November 1982.

Index